A PROFESSION OF ONE'S OWN

Organized Medicine's Opposition to Chiropractic

Susan L. Smith-Cunnien

University Press of America,® Inc.
Lanham • New York • Oxford

Copyright © 1998 by
University Press of America,® Inc.
4720 Boston Way
Lanham, Maryland 20706

12 Hid's Copse Rd.
Cummor Hill, Oxford OX2 9JJ

Library of Congress Cataloging-in-Publication Data

Smith-Cunnien, Susan L.
A profession of one's own : organized medicine's opposition to
chiropractic / Susan L. Smith-Cunnien.
p. cm.
Includes index.
1. Medicine—United States—History—20th century. 2.
Chiropractic—United States—History—20th century. 3.
Professions—United States—Sociological aspects. 4.
Interprofessional relations—United States. 5. American Medical
Association. I. Title.
R152.S58   1997   610'.973'0904—dc21   97—38181 CIP

ISBN 0-7618-0943-0 (cloth: alk. ppr.)

♾™ The paper used in this publication meets the minimum
requirements of American National Standard for information
Sciences—Permanence of Paper for Printed Library Materials,
ANSI Z39.48—1984

To my parents
Mary Roberta and Samuel Penn Smith

Contents

Abbreviations

AAFP	American Association of Family Practitioners
AAPS	Association of American Physicians and Surgeons
ACA	American Chiropractic Association
AHA	American Hospital Association
AMA	American Medical Association
AMAN	American Medical Association News
AMN	American Medical News
BMSJ	Boston Medical and Surgical Journal
CCE	Council on Chiropractic Education
CHB	Chiropractic Health Bureau
HMO	Health maintenance organization
ICA	International Chiropractors Association
JAMA	Journal of the American Medical Association
ME	Medical Economics
NEJM	New England Journal of Medicine
NCHCAC	National Chiropractic Health Care Advisory Committee
ob-gyns	Obstetricians-Gynecologists
PPO	Preferred provider organization
UCA	Universal Chiropractors Association

Preface

J. Stuart Moore described Walter I. Wardwell's recent work on chiropractic history as "yeoman's labor" and described the book itself as a workhorse among books. In the context of scholarship on chiropractic, that comment is high praise indeed. So little of chiropractic history has been documented and so much of what is documented remains unanalyzed that Wardwell's thorough compendium was exactly what was needed.

I see my work here as yeoman's service and should someone describe this book as a workhorse, I will be only too pleased. The medical opposition to chiropractic was, and still is, central to the understanding of the development of chiropractic. Indeed some have argued that had it not been for the rallying effect of medical opposition, chiropractic might not have survived. But nowhere has this opposition been fully documented. In this book I have analyzed why and how the American Medical Association and other medical associations communicated this opposition to chiropractic to its members. I have documented this opposition editorial by editorial, article by article, and news item by news item. What remains for other researchers and future books is a similarly comprehensive documentation of the actions that comprised this opposition and the documentation and analyses of medical opposition to chiropractic in local arenas. This book is a start; much more work remains.

But it would be a mistake to proceed as if the study of organized medicine's opposition to chiropractic is of interest only to chiropractors or that this study is relevant only to the understanding of chiropractic history and progress. Indeed, the premise of this book is that the opposition to chiropractic is an important part -- an integral part -- of medical history as well. Medicine's opposition to chiropractic is part of its effort to claim its status as "a profession of its own."

Physicians often presume that organized medicine's opposition to chiropractic was based solely on the belief that chiropractic theory was erroneous. In this view, physicians opposed chiropractic on scientific grounds. But this view cannot explain why opposition to chiropractic varied so much across the twentieth century. To understand this variation, it is necessary to look at the social functions that opposition to chiropractic provided for organized medicine.

It is a fascinating story. And it is a story that can be fully understood only through the interpretive lens of sociology. There is no conspiracy here. There is only -- and truly -- the realization of how the social dynamics spawned by the opposition of one medical group to another contributed to the development of both.

Acknowledgements

The late Harold Finestone, Gary Alan Fine and Theodor Litman provided much appreciated encouragement and assistance when I began this book, as a dissertation, in graduate school. Thanks, too, to Joachim Savelsberg.

In the intervening years I have been grateful for the support of friends and family, especially my husband, Phil, who went far past his marital obligations by carefully proofing the entire manuscript.

I very much appreciate the cheerful professionalism of the staff at the University Press of America, Inc.

Many thanks to the organizations listed below for their permission to use the copyrighted material noted.

Passages from the following have been reprinted with permission from the *ACA Journal of Chiropractic:* Mark Goodin, "What's a Politician to Think? The Mantra of Primary Care and One Lobbyist's Dilemma," January 1994, Volume 31, No. 1, pages 19-21; "ACA Embarks on Emergency National Mobilization Campaign," January 1993, Volume 30, No. 1, pages 26-29; "R. Reeve Askew, DC, Testifies as Panel Member Before President's Health-Care Task Force," May 1993, Volume 30, No. 5, page 71; "ACA Testifies Before Stark Health-Care Panel," July 1993, Volume 30, No. 7, pages 41, 101; "National Health-Care Reform: ACA Set to Launch Phase

III of Emergency Mobilization Plan," July 1993, Volume 30, No. 7, pages 56-57; Greg Lammert, "ACA's National Chiropractic Legislative Conference Draws Top Government Leaders," April 1994, Volume 31, No. 4, pages 54-61.

Passages from the following have been reprinted with permission from the *Journal of the American Medical Association:* "Medical News-Oregon," February 18, 1928, Volume 90, No. 7, page 553; "Medical News-Massachusetts," November 14, 1931, Volume 97, No. 20, page 1472; Excerpts from Dr. Edward Cary speech in "Council on Medical Education and Hospitals,"April 10, 1937, Volume 108, No. 15, page 1284; "Medicolegal Abstracts - Medical Practice Acts: Chiropractic as the Practice of Medicine," April 22, 1939, Volume 112, No. 16, page 1633; "Current Comment," March 30, 1940, Volume 114, Number 13, page 1270; "Editorial - What Chiropractic is Really Like!" August 6, 1960, Volume 173, No. 14, page 1582; "Letter to the Editor- Answer," March 4, 1961, Volume 175, No. 9, page 833; "Editorial - Chiropractic As a Career," November 23, 1964, Volume 190, No. 8, page 772; "AMAgrams," July 25, 1966, Volume 197, No. 4, page 9.

Passages from the following have been reprinted with permission from the *International Review of Chiropractic:* November/December 1993, Volume 49, No. 6, pages 15-17; "President's Message," September/October 1993, Volume 49, No. 5, pages 7-8; "President's Message," November/December 1993, Volume 49, No. 6, page 9; November/December 1993, Volume 49, No.6, pages 11-13; "President's Message," November/December 1994, Volume 50, No. 6, pages 9-10.

Chapter 1

Introduction: The Development of Medicine and the Battle Against Chiropractic

Chiropractic recently celebrated the centennial anniversary of its discovery in 1895 by D.D. Palmer. Chiropractors throughout the United States -- indeed, from all over the world -- descended upon Davenport, Iowa, the birthplace of chiropractic, to celebrate the survival of their practice. The outlook for chiropractic is rosy today, but this was not always true. Many of the centennial festivities paid homage to those who struggled against the odds, who struggled to survive, throughout most of those one hundred years. In the eyes of most chiropractors, the "odds" against which they were struggling were posed by organized medicine.

As we shall see, it is quite true that organized medicine opposed chiropractic for most of the past century. The question is: Why? Physicians respond that their opposition stems from the inadequacy of chiropractic theory and the lack of evidence supporting both the theory and practice of chiropractic. Chiropractors -- and many social scientists -- respond that medical opposition stems from the fear of chiropractic as an economic competitor. Both of these perceptions may well be true in part. But I argue that neither of these explanations is complete, for neither is able to explain the tremendous variations in the vigor with which chiropractic was opposed across the century. In order to understand this variation, it is necessary to understand the social process of opposition to chiropractic and the role this plays in the development of medicine as a profession. This, then, is a story about medicine more than it is a story about chiropractic, and the story revolves around this notion of "profession."

What are professions? How do they differ from other occupations? Howard Becker (1962) notes that sociologists have often utilized member or "common sense" conceptualizations of professions to differentiate them from other occupations. This approach is theoretically fruitless, he says, and instead defines professions as "those occupations which have been fortunate enough in the politics of today's world to gain and maintain possession of that honorific title" (Becker 1962, pp. 32-33). This title is of concrete importance, however, in that it provides justification and legitimation for the autonomy of occupational groups over their work. It thus becomes a "prize" which many aspiring professions seek.

This basic insight represented a great leap forward in the discussion surrounding the development of professions and the growth of occupational power, for it reintroduced the Hughesian idea that "professions" are socially constructed entities and reminded us of the centrality of politics in this construction process (Hughes 1958, 1965). The analysis of professions and professionalization moved forward quickly in the years after Becker's observations. His view of profession as a symbolic prize with certain desirable consequences provided a beginning point for those working from a conflict or power perspective who eventually asked: What are the conditions under which occupations have the power to successfully stake a professional claim?

But certain basic issues remained relatively untouched in the ensuing discussion and research. What happens in the process of this quest for the professional prize? If we assume that the struggle for the professional prize is in fact a contest rather than a solitary quest, of what import are the actions of other, possibly competing, groups? In striving to reach the "prize" themselves, how might one occupation limit the success of another occupation? What factors influence the selection and direction of such activities? How does the changing structural position of an occupation relate to changes in its status-seeking activities?

These questions are the focus of this book. To answer them I will examine the relations between organized medicine and chiropractic in the United States from the beginnings of chiropractic in 1895 to 1976, the year chiropractors filed a major antitrust suit against the American Medical Association and other medical groups and individuals.[1] After the 1976 lawsuit virtually all public condemnation of chiropractic by organized medical groups ceases. However, I will consider the participation of organized medicine and chiropractic in the health care reform efforts of 1993 and 1994 in order to illustrate how the current situation compares to the past. The focus of the book is really organized medicine. I look at how organized medicine attempts to define itself as a "profession" while defining chiropractic as "quackery" and how changes in the structural position of medicine relate to changes in its definitional activities vis-a-vis chiropractic. I identify three distinct periods in these deviance construction activities and argue that these variations are directly linked to medicine's varying quest for unity, status and dominance throughout this century. My basic argument is that the construction of chiropractic as "quackery" is an integral element of the development of medicine as a profession.

THE DEVELOPMENT OF MEDICINE AND THE CONSTRUCTION OF CHIROPRACTIC AS DEVIANT

Research on occupations often treats the development of professional autonomy and control as a process that takes place in a vacuum, independent of other occupations. When other occupations are considered, interoccupational relations are primarily analyzed in terms of competition for market domination. I propose that there is another aspect of the relations between occupations that is part of the attempt to establish professional autonomy and control: the definitional contest in which occupations attempt to secure favorable definitions of themselves (such as "profession") and unfavorable definitions of other occupations (such as "quackery"). Obviously the standing of each group in this definitional contest has consequences for the occupation's ability to control their environment and their own destiny. After all, definitions which received state support are embodied in the law. The outcome of the definitional contest thus has a direct bearing on the competition for market domination.

But the process of this collective definition must itself be examined, for research in the field of deviance suggests that this process is a central element of the social dynamics of the group. The process of the collective definition of deviance can serve to increase solidarity among the definers when something threatens that solidarity. Importantly, the group or action that is defined as deviant need not be the source of that threat. This perspective provides a broader understanding of the quest for the professional prize.

I argue here that organized medicine, representing the profession of medicine,[2] never considered chiropractic to be a threat. At different points in history medicine considered chiropractic to be an outrage, an irritant, or an enemy, but never really a threat to its domination of the medical arena and certainly never a threat to its survival. However, by collectively opposing chiropractic, organized medicine was able to secure the unity and demonstrate the status necessary to initially foster and later retain professional autonomy and control. Chiropractic itself was not perceived as a threat to orthodox medicine, but the collective definition of chiropractic as deviant enabled medicine to more successfully face the threats it *did* perceive.

To understand organized medicine's construction of chiropractic as a deviant practice and chiropractors as deviant practitioners it is necessary to see this construction process as an integral element of the development of medicine during this century. When I use the term "the development of medicine," of course, I am referring not to the scientific and technological achievements of medicine but rather to the social aspects of orthodox medicine as an occupation: the status of the occupation, the organization of the profession and its professional associations, its relationship with other healing occupations, and its relationship with the state. Superficially, it might appear that the development of medicine has been unilinear -- with progressively higher status, increasingly organized, dominant and autonomous -- but medical historians and sociologists have documented significant variations from this model, particularly during the last thirty years (Starr 1982; Burnham 1982). These changes in the social organization of medicine have influenced the manner in which organized medicine has pursued the social construction of chiropractic as quackery.

MEDICINE VIEWS CHIROPRACTIC: VARIATIONS IN ACTIVE OPPOSITION

If one were to examine the perceptions of organized chiropractic and organized medicine regrading the history of their relations, I suspect both groups would see this history as one of constant opposition to chiropractic by orthodox medicine. For example, physician Joseph Sabatier, in a 1969 editorial in the *Journal of the American Medical Association* (JAMA), states:

Medicine and the scientific community have contended since chiropractic's birth in 1895 that it is an unscientific cult whose practitioners lack the necessary training and education to diagnose and treat human disease.[3]

Likewise, in their monograph *What Medicine Really Thinks about Chiropractic*, chiropractors Weiant and Goldschmidt state:

The dominant tone of medical reaction to chiropractic has always been that of contempt or indignation (1966, p.7).

Sociological analyses of the macro-level process of defining deviance likewise often either assume constancy in the efforts to create deviants (variations being then due to the political success and failures of these efforts) or else examine this process in linear terms (e.g., progressive criminalization, progressive decriminalization, progressive medicalization, and so forth).

Yet an analysis of the data I collected clearly shows that the deviance construction activity of organized medicine vis-a-vis chiropractic has varied in intensity -- both in substance and quantity -- from the early 1900s through 1976. This activity has not varied in a linear fashion. Rather, analysis reveals three rather distinctive periods in the posture taken by the American Medical Association (AMA) vis-a-vis chiropractic. The first period runs from 1908, the year in which chiropractic is first mentioned in JAMA, to 1924 and is characterized by an increasing awareness of chiropractic and increasing deprecation of these practitioners. I call this period "Chiropractic as Outrage" to capture the dual characteristics of incredulity and alarm that characterize this stage in the construction of chiropractic as deviant. The second period encompasses the years 1925 to 1960, a period of consistent but less vituperative opposition to chiropractic. I call this period "Chiropractic as Irritant" to capture the persistent negative but low-level response towards chiropractic during most of this period. The third period covers the years 1961 to 1976 and is characterized by a more offensive stance towards chiropractic. I call this period "Chiropractic as Enemy" to capture the military spirit with which organized medicine battles chiropractic during this period. These periods are not totally homogenous and there are several themes which appear throughout the century. But the distinct differences in medicine's posture toward chiropractic in each of these three periods are quite clear and it is essential to recognize these differences if we are to understand how the deviantization of chiropractic plays a central role in the professional development of medicine in the United States.

ORGANIZATION OF THE BOOK

The book is basically organized along chronological lines. Chapter 2 is an overview of the history of medicine and chiropractic in the United States, providing background and context for the discussion of these two professions. In chapters 3, 4, and 5, the relationship between the changes in the social organization of medicine and medical opposition to chiropractic are documented, with each of the chapters corresponding to one of the periods identified above. Chapter 3 covers the early years 1908 to 1924 where chiropractic first comes to the attention of organized medicine is viewed as an outrage. Chapter 4 covers 1925 to 1960, years during which chiropractic is perceived by organized medicine to be an irritant of sorts. Chapter 5 covers the years 1961 to 1976, years during which organized medicine actively battles chiropractic as the enemy.

In 1976 chiropractors sued the American Medical Association (and others) for violating antitrust regulations. After that point, organized medicine no longer publicly condemned chiropractic. After 1976, then, it is not possible to do the same type of analysis of medical opposition to chiropractic that was done in chapters 3 through 5. Instead, chapter 6 covers the participation of both organized medicine and chiropractic in the recent health reform efforts (1993 to 1994) with the emphasis on how changes in the social organization of medicine and chiropractic are reflected in their participation in the reform process.

Chapter 7 returns to the original questions posed about the process of the development of professions. Here I link the knowledge gained from the study of medicine's opposition to chiropractic to other sociological work in this area, particularly in terms of extending previous analyses of the targets and timing of the deviantization process and how this process may be part of the process of professionalization. Chapter 8, the conclusion, examines how the study of medicine's opposition to chiropractic contributes to the study of deviance and the study of professions.

Scientific questions regarding the therapeutic efficacy of chiropractic and orthodox medical treatments lie outside the scope of sociological analysis and will not be addressed in this book. Any discussion of treatment issues herein is related to public, medical or chiropractic perceptions of efficacy and the social legitimation of chiropractic or medical treatments as effective or ineffective.

NOTES

1. The suit, *Wilk et al vs. AMA et al*, was brought by Chester A. Wilk and four other chiropractors against the AMA and ten other medical associations and five individuals in 1976 (Complaint #76C37777, United States District Court for the Northern District of Illinois, Eastern Division). The chiropractors argued that the AMA and others had violated antitrust laws in conspiring to monopolize medicine. The AMA was found not guilty in 1981, but the court ruled in favor of the chiropractors in subsequent appeals in 1987 and 1990 (Nos. 87-2672 and 87-2777, United States

Court of Appeals for the Seventh Circuit, February 7, 1990).

2. Throughout the book I will frequently use language that appears to reify the concepts of group, occupation and organized medicine by referring to the behavior of occupations and groups in terms such as "the occupation attempts to...." I use such phraseology as shorthand. When I refer to the behavior of the occupation or group I am generally referring to the structured pattern of interactions of the group members or the group leaders.

I use the term organized medicine to refer to the formal association in which physicians have collectively organized themselves. I focus almost exclusively on the American Medical Association (AMA) and its constituent state and local medical societies. I discuss the issue of the AMA as representative of physicians in the U.S. in the methodological appendix, appendix A.

3. JAMA Sept. 15, 1969, 209(11):1712.

Chapter 2

A Brief Social History of Medicine and Chiropractic

To understand the dynamics between organized medicine and chiropractic across this century requires an appreciation of the very different histories of these two professions. As we will see, there are both striking differences and notable similarities in the social pasts of medicine and chiropractic. While it would be too great a generalization to say that throughout the century medicine could look at chiropractic and see an image of itself a decade or two before, this is actually quite true in some respects. In the second decade of this century, for example, when medicine sharply criticized the inadequacies of chiropractic education, it was only a few years from these inadequacies itself. Likewise, medicine today can look at the chiropractor who is likely to work on a fee-for-service basis as a solo practitioner and recognize that as their own dominant form of practice a decade or two ago. With the exception of educational practices, chiropractic has generally changed much less over the century than has medicine.

This chapter will outline the significant events and changes in the history of both chiropractic and medicine. The focus will be on the social aspects of these professions, looking primarily at issues such as the organization of their work, educational institutions, and professional associations. These histories will be presented rather unevenly -- that is, events that appear to have important consequences for the relations between these two groups will be dealt with in greater detail than those events that are not as directly relevant to these relations. Chiropractic began in 1895, so that date will be the starting point of this history. I will begin the history of medicine at a slightly earlier date in order to present a better picture of medicine at the time chiropractic enters the health care arena.

MEDICINE IN AMERICA IN THE NINETEENTH AND TWENTIETH CENTURIES

During most of the nineteenth century, medicine in the United States was quite different from medicine as we know it today. It was different in terms of medical practices and techniques, the organization of service delivery and the professional organization of practitioners. I will discuss each of these dimensions -- along with several other issues of historical and sociological significance -- in the following sections.

Medical Practices and Techniques

During the first half of the nineteenth century much of medical practice was characterized by the so-called "heroic" measures which we now look back upon with horror. The bloodletting practices of lancing and cupping and the application of leeches, the blistering, the administration of powerful emetics and cathartics -- all of these practices reflected the current understandings of disease origins at the time.

By mid-century, the use of these heroic medical practices was starting to be replaced by therapeutic nihilism, on the one hand, and the development of numerous medical sects, on the other. Therapeutic nihilism represented the recognition that current medical practices were causing more harm than good and a recognition of the self-limiting nature of most diseases (Shryock 1974, p. 249). The proliferation of medical sects reflected a number of developments.

The growth of medical sects has been attributed in part to the Jacksonian emphasis on freedom, individualism, and anti-elitism (Shryock 1967, p. 31; 1974, p. 262). Sects like the Thomsonians, for example, emphasized that every person could in effect be their own doctor, using preparations composed of herbs and other natural ingredients. Grahamites emphasized the curative effects of wheat bran foods (such as the "graham cracker") (Deutsch 1977). Other sects that were popular at this time promoted water cures, Hauser's blended vegetable drinks, and magnetic healing. The practitioners of these sects had little or no education or training, typically having only a short course or "home study" course of reading in the techniques and practices of the sect. The Thomsonians trained in "Friendly Botanical Society" meetings, where techniques and preparations were discussed informally (Ehrenreich and English 1978). As Shryock notes (1967, p. 37), much of the superiority of what was known as "regular" medicine at this time stemmed not from any therapeutic superiority but from the higher level of general education of its leaders.

The sects also developed in part as a reaction to the harsh heroic measures of the regular medical practitioners. Not only did many of the sects allow for self- or friend/relation-healing, but the therapeutics offered were much more gentle in their application and effects. Perhaps the major rival to regular medical practitioners during the nineteenth century were the Homeopaths (Kaufman 1971). Homeopathy was started in the late 1700s by Samuel Hahnemann. Homeopathy was dominated by the principals of similars and infintessimals: that illnesses were best attacked by substances that produced states similar to the illness state (rather than trying to engender the opposite state) and that very diluted doses of medications were much more powerful than strong doses of the same medicine. Homeopathy was practiced by homeopathic physicians who underwent much of the same training that regular physicians experienced. Thus, from the patients perspective, homeopathy offered the status of a trained practitioner without having to undergo the frightening course of treatment offered by the regular physician. Perhaps the same could be said for the Eclectics, who utilized a variety of therapeutic modalities, as their name implies, and were also relatively well-trained.

By 1860 most regular practitioners had abandoned the "worst features" of heroic medicine (Berman 1978, p. 79). Advances in bacteriology and surgery, along with changes in hospitals, specialties, and medical education (which will be discussed in later sections), while at first encouraging the therapeutic nihilism mentioned above, gradually gave regular practitioners a therapeutic advantage over many of the medical sects. In the mid-1800s European physicians and researchers, such as Semmelweiss and Snow, had begun to find empirical links between decaying matter or organisms and disease in their studies of childbed fever and cholera. In the 1870s Koch and Pasteur isolated and identified microbes associated with particular diseases.

Major advances in surgery began after Lister began to apply Pasteur's findings regarding the role of microbes in fermentation to the surgical arena with the concept of antisepsis and then asepsis. Although Lister first published in the late 1860s, his ideas were not generally accepted among American surgeons until around 1880 (Earle 1969). The development of effective anesthetics also did much to advance the practice of surgery.

The gradual acceptance of the germ theory of disease had enormous consequences for the practice of medicine. The development and mass administration of vaccines and the encouragement of sanitation and other public health measures (sewage disposal, rational quarantines, etc.) during the 1890s and early decades of the 1900s resulted in vast improvements in public health. Mortality rates had already apparently begun to fall before the acceptance of germ theory, however, due to improvements in nutrition and sanitation efforts that were based on other theories of disease etiology (McKinlay and McKinlay 1977).

Technological advances throughout the nineteenth century allowed for the development of numerous medical instruments which also improved the practice of medicine, primarily by improving diagnostic capabilities. The stethoscope was developed in 1819, the ophthalmoscope in 1851, and the x-ray machine in 1895. Medical specialties frequently began after the development of new instruments.

The development of antibiotics on a mass scale -- sulfa drugs in the 1930s and penicillin in the 1940s -- marked perhaps the next big development in the advancement of public health. Since the 1930s, advances in medicine have continued at a rapid pace. With much of the acute and episodic diseases associated with infection now under control, medical practitioners and researchers currently face the chronic, long-term illnesses that plague an aging population: heart disease, cancer, high-blood pressure and other such illnesses.

Medical Education

The issue of medical education is an important one not only because it has been a central focus in the change of orthodox medicine but also for its role in the increasing differentiation of orthodox medicine from alternative healing occupations. In the early years of medicine in the United States, medical practitioners were trained in one of two ways: either by attending high school, perhaps some college, and a European medical school or by apprenticing oneself to a practicing physician, with the latter form of medical education being the more common. With the onset of medical licensing legislation in the late 1700s and early 1800s, however, there was a shift towards increased numbers of physicians being trained in medical schools. Much of the new licensing legislation gave control over entry to the medical profession to medical societies, which tended to favor formal medical education. Thus entry to the profession became somewhat easier if one was in possession of a medical school diploma. As a result of this, medical schools began to spring up everywhere. Many were of dubious quality and some were merely "diploma mills." The numbers of physicians rose dramatically during the 1800s and by the end of the century physicians noted that there were more regular physicians -- and irregular practitioners, as sect practitioners were sometimes called -- than the market could support (Burrow 1977).

The American Medical Association was formed in 1848 and had as one of its primary goals the improvement of medical education in the United States. Even the best medical schools, such as Pennsylvania and Harvard, which had begun operating in the 1700s and were modeled after the famous European medical schools at Edinborough and Leyden, provided a relatively limited form of education. Most instruction was lecture-based, with few laboratories and little clinical training. By the end of the 1800s, however, there was a push to change medical education in the U.S. to make it more like the German system. The founding of the medical school at Johns Hopkins University in 1893 represented the beginning of this change. Faculties at medical schools changed in that it became desirable for them to be full-time faculty and researchers and to minimize their private practice of medicine. Heretofore most medical school faculties were composed of part-time instructors who were paid directly by the students and who had a competitive advantage over other practitioners since they had access to a patient base by virtue of their connection with the medical schools. The laboratory and clinical components of medical education were expanded. The entrance requirements for these new medical schools were also increased. Schools like Johns Hopkins began to require four years of college, including a basic science background, and knowledge of a foreign language before admittance.

By the early 1900s the American Medical Association (AMA) was pushing strongly for improvement of medical education. In 1907 the AMA instituted a system of classifying the medical schools into three categories. The lowest category of schools were urged to close their doors. Some suggest that the AMA was interested in closing down some of the medical schools not only to improve the quality of physicians but also to reduce the number of physicians (controlling the entry to the profession being one way to control the market) (Burrow 1977).

In 1910 the famous Flexner Report on the state of medical education in the United States was issued. The report was instrumental in the closing of numerous medical schools that existed at its issue. However, a significant number of schools (35 out of 161) had already closed in the years just prior to the release of the report.

In the early 1900s there were a number of other significant developments that influenced medical education. Of primary importance, perhaps, was the changing nature of the hospital. Hospitals during the 1700s and 1800s did not play the same role in medical care that they do today. Hospitals were places where the poor sick were kept or where people went to die. Prior to the acceptance of germ theory and the practice of asepsis, hospitals were dirty places where rampant infections were common. Patients who could afford it were treated at home, even for surgical procedures. Hospitals were utilized in providing some clinical experience for medical students, but not to the extent that they are used today. (And from the perspective of the hospital, hospitals did not depend on the labor of medical students and recent graduates as they do today.)

As knowledge about disease transmission grew and hospitals became safer, more patients were willing to be treated there, providing a larger pool of "learning experiences" for medical students. Just as importantly, however, changes in medical technology during the next few decades (and even more so today) played an important role in the development of hospitals and their place in the system of medical care that we see today. New technologies frequently involved the use of expensive equipment for diagnostic and treatment purposes. While few individual practitioners could afford this equipment, hospitals could purchase it for collective use. Some medical schools had had formal links to hospitals in the 1800s, but in the early 1900s these affiliations became standard. Medical education required training in the use of these new technologies.

Changes in medical education were also related to the influx of funding for such education and for medical research by private foundations beginning in the early 1900s. Between 1910 and the 1930s these foundations poured $300 million into this cause. The General Education Board, a Rockefeller philanthropy, alone contributed over $82 million for medical education reform by 1930 (Brown 1979, p. 193).

Although the American Medical Association was very opposed to any federal funding of medical education in the first decades of the twentieth century -- fearing the potential for government interference in medical education -- after World War II the AMA changed its stance and was willing to accept federal dollars. Today medical schools are substantially subsidized by the federal government, such that 60% of all money spent by medical schools is federally-funded (Brown 1979, p. 227).

Medical Specialization

During most of the history of modern medicine there was very little specialization within the ranks of practicing physicians. With the exception of surgery -- which was as likely to be done by non-physicians such as barbers or by a distinct group of people designated as surgeons but with lower status than general physicians -- there was little specialization. Indeed, during the second half of the 19th century the AMA tried to restrict specialization in practice, rejecting "the claims of scientific leaders that specialism was based on greater expertise not available to the general practitioner" (Brown 1979, p. 93). Specialization that did occur tended to be based on the preference of physicians to treat certain illnesses or patients and the accumulation of expertise on the basis of experience and not on any special medical training in the area. This pattern of specialization was predominant until the 1940s (Hall 1946).

As indicated earlier, developments in technology often preceded the development of certain specialties. Among the first specialty professional organizations, for example, was the society for ophthalmologists, which began in the 1850s shortly after the development of the ophthalmoscope. Other specialties developed in the wake of certain events. For example, Physical Medicine began as an area of medical specialization after World War I, with the influx of the war-injured.

During the twentieth century, medical practice became increasingly specialized. By 1963 general practitioners comprised only 28% of non-federal physicians in the U.S. and by 1973 only 18% (Brown 1979, P. 215). Today even Family Practice is considered a specialty area within medicine.

History of the American Medical Association

This history of the AMA will be fairly general in focus. Materials that relate specifically to AMA relations with chiropractic will be covered in later chapters. A general discussion of the development of the Association and the matters with which it concerned itself is necessary to provide the background for later analysis.

The AMA was founded in 1847. The object of the Association was to raise the quality of medical education and to bar unqualified practitioners from the practice of medicine (Burrow 1963, p. 1; Fishbein 1947, p. 31). A primary objective was to eliminate the sectarian practitioners of medicine in the United States. In 1855 the newly formed organization was already urging the medical profession not to support schools that mixed homeopathy and regular medicine and was encouraging state and local medical societies not to admit sectarians (Burrow 1963, pp. 5-6).

During the years between 1859 and 1900, the AMA exerted much less influence over the course of medical practice and care than in the years since. Although the AMA began publishing its *Transactions* in 1848 and started the Journal of the *American Medical Association* (JAMA) in 1883, these publications had a relatively low subscription audience. As late as 1900, JAMA was received by fewer than one-seventh of the practitioners in the United States (Burrow 1963, p. 14). Early membership in the organization was also small relative to the number of practicing physicians. In the first years of the organization membership was quite exclusive and was limited to delegates from state and local medical societies. However, efforts to increase the numbers and representativeness of AMA membership soon began. In 1862, the AMA began to admit members "by application" so that physicians who were not delegates of medical societies (especially in areas where such societies did not yet exist) could join the Association. However, the AMA sought an enlarged membership only among the regular physicians, not the homeopaths, eclectics, or other irregular practitioners. In 1870, for example, the AMA threatened that it would not admit delegates from the Massachusetts Medical Society unless this society eliminated homeopaths from its membership (which it did) (Kett 1968, p. 29).

In 1901 a major reorganization of the AMA and its relations with constituent societies took place. In the new federalized scheme, local medical societies sent delegates to state medical societies which in turn sent delegates to sit in the House of Delegates of the AMA in proportion to the medical population in the state. The House of Delegates conducted the business of the association, as it does today.

The AMA efforts at unifying the medical profession and establishing a favorable public image took place on many fronts, a few of which will be listed below as illustrations. The AMA's Bureau of Legal Medicine and Legislation sent out information to state and local societies about legislation pending in that state and included the AMA position on that legislation. The AMA also began to provide editorials for state society journals, "canned" speeches for radio broadcasts or public speaking engagements, public relations pamphlets, a speakers bureau, and in 1913 established a Cooperative Medical Advertising Bureau, as a service to state medical society journals to handle the procurement of advertising in their pages (Garceau 1941; Hyde and Wolff 1954; Burrow 1963). In 1927, the AMA started sending a member of the Bureau of Legal Medicine to Washington,

D.C. to remain while Congress was in session. After 1939, AMA efforts to advance their interests were no longer on an *ad hoc* basis (Hyde and Wolff 1954, p. 1010). In 1945, the AMA hired a public relations firm to advise them in public relations matters.

Although it appears clear that a high degree of unity was achieved among the membership of the AMA, it is important to note that divisions among the membership did and do occur. In fact, in the 1930s specific efforts were made to mask dissension and put forth an image of unity.[1] It is clear that certain groups and individuals within the AMA have opposed AMA policy (Garceau 1941). These divisions notwithstanding, the AMA continued to grow throughout most of this century. Garceau reports that 50% of all U.S. physicians belonged to the AMA in 1912, 60% in 1922 and 66.8% in 1940.[2] A decline in membership began in the 1960s. In 1982 the AMA had 251,745 members, representing 45% of all U.S. physicians (Campion 1984). The AMA today, with a membership of about 300,000, continues to represent fewer than half of all physicians.

CHIROPRACTIC IN AMERICA IN THE TWENTIETH CENTURY

Chiropractic began in 1895 with the first chiropractic spinal manipulation by D.D. Palmer in Davenport, Iowa. B.J. Palmer, his son, is credited with establishing the profession. Unlike the dramatic changes in medicine that have occurred during the 20th century -- both in technology and the social organization of medicine -- chiropractic has undergone relatively little change (with the exception of chiropractic education).

Chiropractic Practices and Techniques

D.D. Palmer believed that disease -- or "dis-ease" as chiropractors sometimes said -- is caused by the subluxation or dislocation of vertebrae in the spinal column. He reasoned that a misaligned vertebrae pressed on the nerves emerging form the spine. This interferes with the transmission of neural impulses throughout the body and thus interferes with health. Particular diseases or discomforts can be traced to the subluxation of particular vertebrae. The treatment of disease thus consists of manipulating the misplaced vertebra back into alignment, allowing the nerve impulses to flow unimpeded.[3] These ideas remain central to the philosophy and practice of chiropractic, although some modifications have been made.

Most chiropractors consider themselves to be primary health care providers. Chiropractic consists of a philosophy of illness and treatment which exists in opposition to orthodox medicine. Using Wardwell's (1963) typology, chiropractors are parallel practitioners. That is, chiropractors do not share the assumptions of orthodox medicine or work under their supervision as do ancillary practitioners (such as nurses). Chiropractors do not limit their attention to specific parts of the body as do limited practitioners (such as dentists). Chiropractors typically do not consider themselves to be back specialists. Rather, they treat the entire gamut of diseases and ailments. Although the majority of chiropractors today do not claim that subluxations of the spine cause all disease, they do argue that misplaced vertebrae may create a body state which is more prone to disease and that adjustment of the misplaced vertebrae will allow the body to more effectively fight disease.

The technique of spinal manipulation -- in particular, the chiropractic "thrust" -- has remained the primary tool of the chiropractor. While there have been controversies regarding the advantages and disadvantages of particular manipulations, such as the "hole-in-one" controversy of the 1930s (regarding the manipulation of the Atlas vertebra), the use of some type of spinal manipulation is the mainstay of the chiropractor. A 1977 survey of chiropractors reported that 100% use spinal manipulation in their practices, performing spinal adjustments an average of 120 times per week (more than twice as frequently as any other technique or service) (von Kuster 1980).

Other techniques and therapeutic modalities have sometimes been used as adjuncts to spinal manipulation. In fact, it was popular for some of the early chiropractic schools to offer two degrees, one in chiropractic and one in naturopathy. This practice had disappeared by the late 1950s (Gibbons 1980). Not all chiropractors have employed adjunct therapies. Chiropractic is divided into two groups, traditionally known as the "straights" and the "mixers". Traditionally, straight chiropractors employed no adjunct therapies. Today chiropractors who employ no adjunct therapies at all are sometimes called "super-straights." Recent data indicates that most chiropractors today employ the following therapies in addition to spinal manipulation: extremity adjustments (employed by 86% of chiropractors surveyed); pressure point or reflex techniques (78%); vitamin/diet supplementation (84%); supports/braces (82%); dietary counseling (84%); exercise counseling (89%); and ultra sound (64%) (von Kuster 1980, pp. 83-84). Other therapies such as massage and low-voltage electrotherapy are used by smaller percentages of chiropractors.

Chiropractic Education

In the first years of chiropractic, chiropractic education consisted of only a few months instruction in the application of chiropractic spinal manipulation. No courses in general biology, physiology, anatomy, bacteriology, or other sciences were included in the curriculum. Students practiced their skills on each other and students with advanced standing refined their skill on patients attending the clinics associated with the chiropractic school. Clinical training in college-sponsored clinics remains an integral part of chiropractic education today. Wardwell (1982, pp. 216-217) reports as an example that "Carver Chiropractic College offered a nine-month course in 1908, an 18-month course in 1910, and a 30-month course in 1930."

By the 1920s the curriculum in many chiropractic colleges included the following subjects: Anatomy, Histology, Physiology, Bacteriology, Pathology, Hygiene and Sanitation as well as chiropractic theory and practice (see, for example, Stanford Research Institute 1960, pp. 92-94). Students were required to attend school for three school years. However, the typical school year lasted only six months, so students could seek employment to pay their expenses and support their families during the off-months.[4] This meant that the chiropractic curriculum was actually only eighteen months (and the "compressed" course was also available).

The "mixer" schools generally included more "medical" training, such as courses in radiography and dissection. Initially, the inclusion of these courses resulted in a great deal of controversy. The decision to offer these courses, of course, had major implications for the definition or view of the nature of chiropractic as a "drugless" healing art that is distinct from orthodox medicine, based on an entirely different approach to the etiology of disease, and to which therefore these more medical courses are irrelevant. It was also seen as a way to raise the status of chiropractic in the eyes of the public and medical practitioners. On the one hand, chiropractors were attempting to differentiate themselves from orthodox practitioners; on the other, they recognized that their poor educational curriculum was one of the major points on which orthodox medicine attacked chiropractic and to the extent that chiropractic education came to "look like" medical education, there would be less basis for attack. These conflicting themes run through the history of chiropractic to the present day.

Changes in the curriculum continued. National College of Chiropractic began offering a 4-year program (of nine months per year) in 1934 and this was the standard chiropractic course by the 1950s (Wardwell 1982).

One aspect of the curriculum that is fairly unique to chiropractic education, in comparison to other healing arts, is the typical inclusion of course work on the business aspect of the occupation: how to establish a clientele, organize an office, and so forth. In the very early years of chiropractic these courses assumed a rather prominent place in the curriculum. Today they constitute a very minor aspect of the curriculum.

The issue of academic requirements for students entering chiropractic schools is another area of both controversy and change. There were almost no prerequisites for students entering the fledgling chiropractic schools. While a significant proportion of the first students did have a strong educational background -- indeed, as Gibbons (1981) has noted, numerous physicians took the course in chiropractic -- most of the students appear to have had only a grade school education.

It was not until the early 1950s that some chiropractic schools began to require some college courses as prerequisites for entrance, although many students did in fact have some college education before attending chiropractic school. For example, the Stanford Research Institute (1960) found that half the students at two California chiropractic colleges had completed one year or more of college study. The first college courses to be required for entrance to chiropractic school were some of the basic science courses such as biology and chemistry.

It is difficult to generalize about early chiropractic educational requirements since there was no single regulatory agency and there was much variation from school to school. John Nugent, the Director of Education for the National Chiropractic Association, established criteria for accreditation in 1941 and the International Chiropractors Association followed suit shortly afterward by establishing its own accreditation commission (Wardwell 1992). In 1974, however, the Council on Chiropractic Education (CCE) was recognized by the U.S. Office of Education as the official accrediting agency for chiropractic colleges. Starting in 1979, the CCE established entrance requirements of a minimum of 2 years of college with a C+ average and at least 4200 classroom hours in the chiropractic program (Commission of Inquiry 1979). Many chiropractic schools had required two years of college course work for entrance earlier in the 1970s. Today the required prerequisite college course work includes anatomy, physiology, two semesters of inorganic chemistry, two semesters of organic chemistry and two semesters of physics. Many chiropractic students today have a college degree prior to entering chiropractic school. Wardwell reports that about half the students entering the better chiropractic colleges enter with a bachelors degree (1982 p. 230). About one-third of the

1988 entering class at Northwestern College of Chiropractic had a college degree (Northwestern College of Chiropractic 1989, p. 24). Today, these percentages are higher, with about 80% of those matriculating in the better chiropractic colleges having a college degree (Wardwell 1992, p. 147).

Chiropractic colleges have differed historically from orthodox medical schools in a number of ways other than curriculum. In the early years of the occupation, the schools were the primary organizational institutions through which chiropractors could (and did) collectively organize themselves. Prior to 1906 there were no professional associations and even when the associations began, they were primarily legal protection associations. The first chiropractic school, the Palmer Institute and Infirmary, was established in 1897 and remained the only school for several years. Shortly afterwards Palmer's students began to establish their own schools. Some students, who by then were teachers at Palmer, developed notions of chiropractic and chiropractic education that conflicted with the Palmer perspective; for example, some wanted more emphasis on dissection and others wanted less emphasis on radiography. These students, such as John Howard, Solon Langworthy, and Oakley Smith, left to start their own schools based on slightly different philosophies and educational methods (Gibbons 1977).

Again, these early schools were the primary organizational affiliation of most chiropractors. Annual homecomings were often very special events that drew large numbers of alumnae. The Palmer School epitomizes this. The school held annual "Lyceums" which were part homecoming gala and part continuing education. The Lyceums also offered a forum for B.J. Palmer to promote his own ideas and chiropractic gadgets (which were leased only through the school at very high rates).

Like the early medical schools in the United States chiropractic schools were proprietary organizations. Although the proprietary medical schools had converted or closed their doors shortly after the release of the Flexner report in 1910, chiropractic schools remained proprietary until 1939 when John Nugent, Director of Education of the National Chiropractic Association, convinced the proprietors of nineteen chiropractic schools to relinquish ownership (Stanford Research Institute 1960). Even after they were no longer privately owned, however, chiropractic schools were funded through student fees and private donations. Chiropractic schools received no federal funds and chiropractic students received no federal assistance until 1974 (with the exception of grants to veterans after World War II).

The number of chiropractic schools in existence has varied across time. Growing from a single chiropractic school in Davenport, Iowa in 1897, there were 17 schools in existence in the U.S. in 1980 (Wardwell 1982); there are

17 today, as well. Several of the schools today have been in existence for over 80 years, although they have sometimes changed their name or location. There have been so many chiropractic schools that opened and closed within a few years that it is difficult to know the precise number of chiropractic schools in existence at any one point in history. However, it appears that there were 79 schools in existence in 1920, 50 schools in existence in 1930, and 20 schools in existence in 1940 (Wardwell 1951). There were 15 schools in existence in 1963 (Gibbons 1977).

The Palmer College of Chiropractic, which teaches "pure" or "straight" chiropractic, is now and has always been the largest of the chiropractic colleges. Although there were only a few students at first, with only fifteen graduates during its first 5 years, it reached a peak enrollment of 3100 in 1922. Thereafter enrollments declined, reaching fewer than 300 in 1929 (Gibbons 1980, p. 19). In 1980 it enrolled 1,826 students (Wardwell 1982). The next largest school is National College of Chiropractic, which teaches broad-scope or "mixer" chiropractic. National was established by John Howard in 1906 in Davenport, moved to Chicago in 1908, and is now located in Lombard, Illinois, a Chicago-suburb. In 1980 National enrolled 878 students (Wardwell 1982). The average enrollment for chiropractic colleges today is 650.

Organization of Chiropractic Practice

Chiropractors today primarily practice as solo practitioners or in practices with one or two other practitioners. A recent survey by the American Chiropractic Association reported that 71% of the respondents were solo practitioners (Plamadon 1993). These figures have remained fairly constant for the last 15 years: a 1977-1979 survey reported that 77% of chiropractors who had been practicing for more than two years were solo practitioners and 9% practiced in groups or partnerships (with an average of 2.5 members) (von Kuster 1980). This, of course, is quite unlike the dramatic changes in practice arrangements among MDs during this same time period. In 1991, only 43% of physicians practiced alone or with one other physician and 33% of physicians practiced in groups (with the rest involved in "other patient care") (AMA 1993). Recent graduates of chiropractic college frequently begin their practice on a salary basis working for another chiropractor and then after a few years leave to set up their own solo practice or form a partnership (von Kuster 1980).

Historically, the dominant mode of practice has been solo practice as well. Although systematic data regarding the organization of practice is not available for the early years of chiropractic practice, all indications are that solo practice was the dominant form. Publications of chiropractors writing during the early period of chiropractic refer only to the single practitioner operating alone, and indeed, the chance to be one's "own boss" was used as a drawing card to attract potential students to chiropractic. Data from California in 1958 show that almost all chiropractic practitioners practiced solo (Stanford Research Institute 1960).

Most of the large chiropractic clinics, both historically and today, were associated with chiropractic colleges. There were few large independent clinics and that remains true today. Part of this, no doubt, is due to the fact that the practice of chiropractic has never required the purchase of expensive technical equipment. Therefore the economic incentive to consolidate practice in order to distribute large capital costs did not exist for chiropractors. The most expensive piece of equipment in most chiropractic offices today is the x-ray machine and not all chiropractors have these (88% of chiropractors indicate they offer some type of x-ray service) (von Kuster 1980, p. 83).

The exception, perhaps, to the predominant mode of solo chiropractic practice was the chiropractic hospital movement of the 1920s and 1930s. In the period from about 1920 to 1940 there were almost one hundred in-patient facilities (Gibbons 1980). The most famous and long lasting chiropractic hospital with its associated clinic was the Spears Chiropractic Hospital in Colorado. Established during World War II, this hospital operated for many years with a capacity of 800-beds, although occupancy declined after the death of founder Leo Spears in 1956 (Gibbons 1980).

It is estimated that in the mid-1970s there were fewer than a dozen in-patient chiropractic facilities in operation (Gibbons 1977). It is not clear why the hospital movement in chiropractic disappeared, although it was no doubt related to three factors: the difficulty for such facilities to receive the necessary licensing from the states; the absence of federal funding to build such facilities; and the lack of insurance (both private and governmental) to cover the expenses of patients utilizing these facilities.[5]

It is difficult to ascertain the precise number of chiropractors who were in practice at various points in the history of chiropractic since this data was rarely collected systematically. Data presented by Wardwell (1982, p. 219) indicates that roughly 100 were in active practice in 1906, 400 to 600 in 1908, 7,000 in 1916, and roughly 16,000 were in practice in 1929. There were about 23,000 practicing chiropractors in 1979 (von Kuster 1980). Estimates reported elsewhere are contradictory. For example, in 1961 the chiropractic associations estimated there were 25,000 practicing DCs The census estimate for 1960 was 14,360 practicing DCs; in 1970 it was 13,729. Meanwhile the National Center for Health Statistics found 17,559 in 1974; and the Federation of Chiropractic Licensing Boards found 29,007 active state chiropractic licenses, but only 17,895 residents licensed to practice chiropractic in 1976 (von Kuster 1980). It appears that up until the 1950s many chiropractic graduates did not engage in active chiropractic practice. Additionally, it appears that many who did actively practice chiropractic did so on a part-time basis (the practice not generating sufficient income). Among California chiropractors in 1958, 77% percent practiced chiropractic more than 32 hours per week (Stanford Research Institute 1960). Among chiropractors today, 90% practice on a full-time basis (more than 30 hours per week) (von Kuster 1980). Today there are about 45,000 practicing chiropractors (ACA 1993).

Chiropractic Specialization

Historically, most chiropractors considered themselves general practitioners. This is generally true today as well, and is especially true for chiropractors who practice pure or straight chiropractic, who sometimes note that the idea of a chiropractic specialist is a contradiction in terms (alluding to the "one cause, one cure" philosophy). Some chiropractors who are broad-scope or mixer practitioners consider themselves specialists. However, these practitioners usually mean that they are a specialized branch of the healing arts, as are podiatrists and internists (Lin 1972, p. 193). For example, in the 1958 survey of California chiropractors, 51% said they were in general practice and 23% said they were specialists in spinal manipulation (Stanford Research Institute 1960).

There apparently has always been some specialization within the practice of chiropractic -- such as practitioners who have large pediatric practices or who specialize in upper cervical cases -- but such specialization of practice is and was not common, usually develops over time as a preference of the practitioner, and is not usually based upon the specialized training of the practitioner. This model of specialization is akin to that of the medical profession in the 1940s as described by Hall (1946). However, patterns of specialization in chiropractic may be changing. Almost 21% of chiropractors have taken some post-graduate study in areas such as nutrition or neurology, but "only about 100 DCS of 23,000 DCS nationally are recognized with Diplomate status from one of the chiropractic associations" (von Kuster 1980, p. 103). Currently, board certification is available from specialty councils of the American Chiropractic Association in seven areas (diagnosis and internal disorders, diagnostic imaging, neurology, nutrition, occupational health, orthopedics, sports injuries and physical fitness) (Wardwell 1992).

History of the Major Chiropractic Associations

In contrast to the medical profession, chiropractic has been much less successful in establishing a unified organizational structure. As noted earlier, chiropractic has been divided into at least two segments almost since its beginning. The controversy between the "straight" and "mixer" chiropractic practitioners was very impassioned in the early years of the occupation. It appears that the fury engendered in this internal strife was equal to that of the external battle with medicine. B.J. Palmer and other straights sometimes referred to mixer chiropractors as "chiropracTOIDS" (sic) or "termites." Mixer chiropractors in turn called B.J. the "Tsar of Chiropractic" and accused him and straight chiropractors of attempting "fratricide."

In 1906 the Universal Chiropractors Association (UCA) was formed in Davenport, Iowa, as an organization whose primary goal was to provide legal assistance to chiropractors charged with practicing medicine without a license. This organization was headed by B.J. Palmer, son of chiropractic's founder D.D. Palmer, until he was expelled (or retired) from the organization in 1925. In 1922, prior to B.J.'s departure from the UCA, the American Chiropractic Association (ACA) split from the UCA partially in response to B.J.'s domination of that organization and his refusal to fully incorporate mixer chiropractors into the organization. Shortly after this point, in 1926, B.J. went on to establish the Chiropractic Health Bureau (CHB), an association of straight practitioners which provided insurance for members. In 1930, the ACA and the declining UCA merged to form the National Chiropractic Association (NCA), which included both straight and mixer chiropractic practitioners (although the mixer practitioners far outnumbered the straights, most of whom were disaffected from B.J. and so not members of the CHB). In 1942, the name of the CHB was changed to the International Chiropractors Association (ICA).[6] B.J. continued to head this organization until his death in 1961, although, as Gibbons (1980, p. 10) notes, he was basically a "titular leader" in this and his other capacities after 1924.

In 1963 there was an attempt to effect a merger between the disparate camps within chiropractic, but on the day in 1964 which the new merger was to be enacted, the ICA failed to send representation. The NCA, disaffected members of the ICA, and other independent practitioners then established the current American Chiropractic Association (ACA). The ICA and the ACA remain as the national professional associations representing the two disparate camps in chiropractic today. However, plans are currently underway to merge these two organizations and it appears possible that the merger may actually take place.

Some dual professional associations exist at the state level as well. Neither the ACA nor the ICA have many formal organizational links to the state and local chiropractic associations, although a few associations are affiliates of one or the other national associations.

As noted earlier, in the early years of chiropractic, the advocates of new positions and those who rejected new developments within existing schools started new schools of chiropractic. Turner (1931, p. 181) notes that these schools "controlled their graduates to an astonishing degree" and that the leaders which emerged from them were very partisan. This decreased the likelihood of chiropractic solidarity.

In the early years of chiropractic (up to 1920 or so), as I noted earlier, these schools were the predominant organizational form within chiropractic. Although the UCA had been established in 1906, it functioned primarily as a legal protection agency and its annual meetings were held at the same time and place as the yearly homecoming of the Palmer School of Chiropractic. Additionally, not all chiropractors belonged to the UCA, which excluded all mixer chiropractors until 1910 and thereafter gradually admitted mixers but offered them only limited protection (Dye 1969, pp. 130-131.) The chiropractic schools were not the functional equivalents of the non-existent, weak, or factionalized professional associations. Yet their existence provided an organizational focus for chiropractors -- practically as well as symbolically -- and the allegiance of alumni, although not blind, was certainly vehement. It is clear that factionalism by school and "school of thought" impeded the development of a single cohesive professional association.

The straight-mixer controversy continued even after local, state, and national associations began to spring up in chiropractic. As noted earlier the opposition between these groups has been and continues to be quite intense. Instances where the straight chiropractors have aligned themselves with medical practitioners in legal battles against mixer chiropractors can be found throughout the history of chiropractic to the present day. For example, in 1938 straight chiropractors supported the Iowa Supreme Court in its affirmation of the injunction against a mixer chiropractor for using physiotherapeutic techniques (Dye 1969). In the late 1960s and early 1970s, attempts to expand the Missouri chiropractic practice law to include the use of light, heat, exercise and other therapies were opposed by the ICA (Lin 1972). In 1980, the president of a straight chiropractic college testified against a Georgia chiropractor who had sued the local school board for not allowing him to conduct the physical exams required for sports participation. Even during the health care reform efforts of the 1990s, as will be discussed in chapter 6, the two major professional associations worked together in an only minimal way. These are but a few examples of chiropractic segmentation in action .

Summary

The differences between orthodox medicine and chiropractic are many: there are differences in therapeutic techniques and practice, differences in education, differences in specialization, and differences in professional organization. Orthodox medicine has undergone tremendous changes in all of these areas in the last one-hundred years. In comparison, there have been fewer changes in chiropractic, with the significant exception of chiropractic education, where change has been very dramatic. The relationship between these and other changes in the histories of medicine and chiropractic and changes in the relations between these two groups will be discussed in later chapters.

NOTES

1. For example, Fishbein reports that in 1931: "Societies of limited membership were requested to refrain from expressing individual and varying opinions. The medical profession should speak, the delegates believed, as a unit rather than present a divided opinion before legislators and the public" (Fishbein 1947, p. 392). Likewise, he reports that in 1932 plans were made to meet with all editors of state periodicals "to unify policies and discuss editorial control of these publications" (Fishbein 1947 p.395). These and other efforts are discussed by Garceau, who refers to this as "the little hoax of unanimity" (1941, p. 73).

2. There may be some disagreement regarding these figures. For example, using data resented in the Appendix of Burrow (1963, pp. 399-400, which are in turn taken from "Report of the Secretary," *JAMA* 74 (May 1, 1920):1233), I calculate that in 1920 there were 44, 992 members of AMA out of 145,384 physicians in the U.S., which is a 31% membership rate. Although it is certainly possible that the membership rate could have doubled to 60% by 1922, it seems more likely that there are some measurement issues that need to be clarified here.

3.   Actually, many chiropractors did not use the word "treatment." They used the word "adjustment," noting that the "innate intelligence" of the body does the healing, not the chiropractor. This choice of words may not have been accidental, since it served as a useful means of avoiding legal prosecution for practicing medicine without a license in the early years of the occupation (Turner 1931).

4.   Unlike medical students during this period who, typically came to medical school directly after graduating from college, chiropractic students tended to be older, self-supporting, and already in the work force for some period of time.

5.   Here one can compare chiropractic with osteopathy, which successfully established numerous hospitals that remained a valuable resource for osteopathy (Albrecht and Levy 1982).

6.   Leis (1971) reports that the ICA was originally the International Chiropractic Congress.

Chapter 3

Medicine Awakens to Chiropractic, 1908-1924: Chiropractic as Outrage

Chiropractic is a freak offshoot from osteopathy. Disease, say the chiropractors, is due to pressure on the spinal nerves; ergo it can be cured by "adjusting" the spinal column. It is the sheerest quackery, and those who profess to teach it make their appeal to the cupidity of the ignorant. Its practice is in no sense a profession but a trade - and a trade that is potent for great harm. It is carried on almost exclusively by those of no education, ignorant of anatomy, ignorant even of the fundamental sciences on which the treatment of disease depends.

Editorial in the *Journal of the American Medical Association*, 1913[1]

These words capture the spirit of the medical profession's reaction to the advent of chiropractic near the turn of the century. Indeed, one can almost hear and feel the sputtering of physicians outraged by the audacity of the new practitioners of chiropractic in editorial after editorial in the major medical publications of the time. These reactions to chiropractic were very much related to the changes that medicine was undergoing at the time. Remember that the latter part of the 19th century and the beginning of the 20th century was a period of rapid change for orthodox medicine in the United States. In terms of the social development of medicine, there were significant changes taking place regarding the status and organization of the profession. First, the American Medical Association (AMA) launched a major campaign to unify the profession organizationally. Second, physicians were trying to increase the social status of medicine. Third, organized medicine was working to secure for orthodox physicians a dominant position with respect to other healing practitioners. The reactions of medicine to chiropractic played an important role in these changes in the organization and status of medicine. Chiropractic provided an impetus for medical unity, a foil for the development of medicine's professional identity, and a way to demonstrate superiority.

This first period of organized medicine's opposition to chiropractic actually begins with very little attention being given to chiropractic. This is no doubt in part due to the fact that chiropractic itself was fairly new, having existed at this point in history for little more than a decade. Although there are indications that chiropractic had spread far from its Iowa origins, the number of chiropractic practitioners was still relatively small. However, in this early part of the first period it appears that, even after acknowledging the existence of chiropractic, the editors of the *Journal of the American Medical Association* (JAMA) and other major medical publications do not really take chiropractic seriously. This can be seen from both the manner in which chiropractic material is presented and the content of that material. In their eyes, chiropractic is simply too outrageous. The initial lack of attention to chiropractic, the routine reporting of chiropractic legal convictions throughout this period, the simple reprinting of others' opinions regarding chiropractic and the reprinting of writings and publications of chiropractors without much additional commentary, as well as the sentiments expressed in these reports, all point to a view of chiropractic as too preposterous to consider seriously. The first entries regarding chiropractic always have the term enclosed in quotation marks or refer to "so-called" chiropractors. Indeed, until 1913 the reports by JAMA staff or other authors do not themselves explicitly criticize or deride chiropractic. After 1913, however, the reaction to chiropractic is clearly one of outrage. Chiropractic is alternately referred to in scathing terms or ridiculed in a humorous fashion.

This chapter will first consider the reaction of medicine to chiropractic, looking at both the way in which material about chiropractic is presented in medical publications and the content of that material. The second part of the chapter will examine the changes occurring in medicine and will link the outrage of medicine toward chiropractic to these changes. For the reader who is interested in looking at information on the amount of material published by several medical publications over the century, this information is available in a variety of tables and figures in appendix B. The focus is on the material relating to chiropractic that is published in JAMA, since this was the preeminent nationally-distributed publication of orthodox medicine, although material in other publications will be noted occasionally.

THE REACTION OF MEDICINE TO CHIROPRACTIC

The Manner of Presentation of Chiropractic-Related Material in Medical Publications

How orthodox medicine refers to chiropractic in medical publications is as telling as the substance of these references. Organized medicine declares its renunciation of chiropractic as outrageous and absurd from the initial lack of attention to chiropractic at all, to the routine reporting of legal convictions of chiropractors, through the practice of reprinting what others have said about chiropractic -- and what chiropractors themselves say -- and the humorous ridicule of chiropractic.

Initial Lack of Attention The entry of chiropractic into the pages of JAMA was quite inauspicious. Although chiropractic began in 1895, there is no mention of chiropractic in JAMA until 1908 and no mention in the *Boston Medical and Surgical Journal* (BMSJ, later to become the *New England Journal of Medicine*) until 1915. In JAMA these first entries are simply brief reports of the conviction of a chiropractor in Iowa for practicing medicine without a license and the defeat of a chiropractic bill in Oklahoma.[2] The three 1909 JAMA entries consist of a reference to the attempt by chiropractors to get legal recognition in several western states, the conviction of a chiropractor for practicing medicine without a license in New York, and the appeals filed by chiropractors (and other "peculiar varieties of applicants") whose licensing applications were refused by the Washington State Board of Medical Examiners.[3] The five items published in 1910 that mention chiropractic are similar in nature with the exception that there is one report from Missouri of a chiropractor who was charged with practicing medicine without a license but successfully used the defense that chiropractors do not use medicine and so do not fall under the medical practice acts.[4] The four 1911 entries regarding chiropractic are all in the "medicolegal" section of the journal and are reports of state Supreme Court decisions affirming the convictions of chiropractors under the medical practice acts in Missouri, Kansas, Washington, and Iowa.[5]

Routine Reporting of Chiropractic Legal Convictions The reports in the "Medicolegal" section of JAMA, which comprise the bulk of the references to chiropractic in the early period, basically point out the facts of the case and the judicial ruling on the case. All cases reported were instances where the courts ruled against the chiropractor in question. This suggests, perhaps, that the journal editors were not really worried about chiropractic establishing itself as an alternative to orthodox medical care.

Reprinting Items with Little Additional Commentary Several references to chiropractic simply reprint quotations from other sources and include little additional comment. These other sources always belittle chiropractors or chiropractic. For example, the first chiropractic-related entry in JAMA in 1908 reprints an editorial from an Oklahoma newspaper that states that the idea that physicians, who are educated, could support a chiropractic bill "is to (sic) absurd to consider."[6] The staff of the "Medical Economics" section, in which this reprint is published, merely adds a congratulatory note to the press for their stance. The next commentary, in 1912, in the section "The Propaganda for Reform," reprints a series of letters between the author and several "so called drugless institutions",[7] one of which is the National School of Chiropractic. Other than an introductory statement of the problem (that various cults are trying to enter medicine through the back door and that the public is not qualified to make distinctions between health practitioners), there is no additional commentary. The reprinted letters are grammatically incorrect letters written by the prospective pseudo-applicant and the responses from the school administrators assure the applicant that they would do well to take the course in chiropractic. These letters are apparently seen as sufficient to make the author's point. This method of reprinting the writings and publications of chiropractors themselves continues through to the present day. However, it was a dominant from of reporting on chiropractic in JAMA in this early period.[8]

The *New England Journal of Medicine* (NEJM) also utilizes the technique of reprinting articles or comments on chiropractic first published elsewhere, but does so to a much lesser degree than does JAMA. For example, a 1921 editorial focuses on a report published in the *New York Times* regarding the deaths of two patients treated by chiropractors (deaths due to appendicitis).[9] A 1923 editorial notes a report in the St. Louis *Star* of a chiropractic diploma mill.[10] Some of these reprints include additional commentary and some do not. For example, the 1921 editorial mentioned above (noting the deaths of the two chiropractic patients) includes what is presumably other information from the *New York Times* article ("Although the parents of the patients were justly alarmed by the cruel manipulations of the chiropractors, they were beguiled by the assertions of the pretenders to procrastinate until too late to bring effective treatment to the sufferers.") and also some editorial warnings ("Massachusetts will be assailed. People should be warned.") and an admonition to readers to refer to articles on the dangers of chiropractic previously published in BMSJ.[11]   Other reprints include no other comments at all. For example, a 1924 reprint from the New York *Tribune* regarding chiropractic attempts at securing legal recognition in New York has no additional commentary.[12]

The implication of these methods of presenting materials appears to be that chiropractors are indeed "too absurd" to consider seriously and that it is sufficient to either quote the opinions of others or to let chiropractors' own writings demonstrate this point.

In the latter part of this early period there is more commentary, although the bulk of JAMA publications regarding chiropractic continue to be medicolegal reports (see table 1 in appendix B). Much of this commentary is directly critical of chiropractic. The substance of this criticism will be discussed later.

Humorous Ridicule   Toward the end of this period, JAMA editors begin to employ humor in their consideration of chiropractic, primarily in the form of humorous ridicule. To some extent, this ridicule continues the format of quoting chiropractors' own writings and the writing of others. I will present a number of examples so the reader can get a sense of the types of comments being published in JAMA at this time.

A 1919 "Current Comment" prints an excerpt from a chiropractic advertising pamphlet that says "...to advertise inside the chiropractic, medical and truth laws, requires some adroitness, some ingenuity of expression, some more than common ability as a wordsmith." To this the editorial adds a final comment: "We'll say it does!"[13]

In 1920 the legal definition of chiropractic passed by the New Jersey state legislature -- a one-hundred-and-forty-six-word sentence -- is reprinted in "Current Comment" with the following commentary:

> Lucidity itself! The New Jersey legislature said "Let there be light on chiropractic" - and, behold, it became the "art of permitting the restoration of the triune relationships between all attributes necessary to normal composite forms, to harmonious quantities and qualities...." Simplicity to the nth power. Bring on your Einstein theory - the New Jersey solons may oblige with a snappy definition.[14]

In February 1921 a short editorial called "Taking Chiropractic Seriously" reprinted the following chiropractic testimonial:

> "Dear Doctor. - Before taking your Chiropractic and Electric treatments, I was so nervous that NOBODY could sleep with me. After taking six treatments ANYBODY can sleep with me."[15] (emphasis in the original)

The editors add that "It would be fatal for a chiropractor to have a sense of humor; in fact, if he had it, he never would have become a chiropractor."[16]

A July 1921 letter to the editor points out that credit for heavy weight boxer Jack Dempsey's victory was given to Nuxated Iron in a previously published comment in JAMA. The writer points out that according to an article in a Des Moines newspaper, the real credit goes to a chiropractor on Dempsey's training staff. The letter, with tongue in cheek, concludes: "I hope you will give credit where it is due."[17]

In September 1921, the issue of veterinary chiropractic is discussed with a sarcastic warning to chiropractors:

> It is one thing to fool with the health of human beings and an entirely different thing to fool with the health of livestock.... That men, ignorant of the body and its processes, should treat the ailments of men, women and children is apparently a small thing; human life is the only thing involved. But that ignoramuses should trifle with he health of a horse or hog is an outrage; that is property. If chiropractors are wise, they will confine their malpractice to humans; it is safer.[18]

This column then inspired another reader to write a letter to the editor about a similar case. A local farmer had a problem with a heifer. When the farmer mentioned the problem in the presence of the chiropractor who was attending his wife, the chiropractor offered to "adjust" the heifer.

> The farmer tells the story and thinks it is a great joke that the chiropractor should attempt to adjust the heifer, but it has not yet dawned on the farmer that there is any joke in the chiropractor adjusting his wife.[19]

In all of these illustrations, chiropractic is ridiculed and treated as a joke. Yet, as the last illustration clearly points out, orthodox practitioners see chiropractic as more than a joke. The very fact that chiropractic is so often the focus of levity in JAMA is, perhaps, revealing in and of itself. Sociologists of humor point out that humor is one method through which uncertainties and ambiguous phenomena can be considered and social definitions can be reached. That certainly appears to be occurring here.

The Substance of Chiropractic-Related Material in Medical Publications

The manner in which material about chiropractic is presented in medical publications clearly demonstrates organized medicine's view that chiropractic is outrageous and absurd. The content of this material declares medicine's reaction to chiropractic even more explicitly.

As noted earlier, there is actually very little original editorial commentary regarding chiropractic in the pages of JAMA during the first half of this period, although there is more such commentary in the last part of the period (after 1920). Yet the commentary, scant as it is, is revealing. Commentary throughout the entire early period is quite derogatory, either directly through vituperative comments or indirectly through humorous ridicule. Chiropractic is routinely referred to as quackery but other derogatory names are frequently used as well. For example, chiropractic is called a "freak off-shoot of osteopathy",[20] the "circus cult",[21] a "menace",[22] and "mountebankery".[23]

There are several themes that run through the medical comments about chiropractic. The 1913 quote that begins this chapter epitomizes the medical reaction to chiropractic so well because it refers to so many of these themes: concern with the poor preparation and training of chiropractors, the inability of the public to judge chiropractic, the continuous provision of information updates on chiropractic, and references to the lower class origins of chiropractors.

The tone of the chiropractic-related items published in NEJM was generally dispassionate, at least in comparison to many of the items published in JAMA. Sometimes the writing appears inflammatory, but for the most part this is not the case. While there are numerous examples of the vilification of chiropractic, as will be presented below, much of the vituperative language consists of a few phrases or sentences in an otherwise "rationally-toned" item. There are almost no completely vituperative diatribes against chiropractors or chiropractic of the intensity seen in the pages of JAMA. The most derogatory articles in NEJM tend to be those published in the 1920s and 1930s,[24] years during which bills to legalize the practice of chiropractic were being considered by the Massachusetts legislature. Although these years are somewhat later than the time period under consideration in this chapter, I include them here because they illustrate the language and themes appearing in JAMA during this earlier period. Chiropractors and chiropractic are referred to in NEJM editorials as "back breakers",[25] a "cult" making "unsound" claims,[26] with a history fraught with "ignorance, sophistry, charlatanism, quackery, fraud".[27] Letters published in the NEJM editorial department refer to chiropractic as "an unintelligent and silly cult"[28] and to "hocus-pocus spine 'adjustments'."[29] Many of the themes about chiropractic that appear in JAMA appear in NEJM as well. It is to these themes we now turn.

Concern with Poor Preparation and Training of Chiropractors From the very first editorial comments about chiropractic in medical publications, the focus on the lack of entrance requirements and the paucity of training involved in chiropractic education is apparent. The 1913 editorial that is quoted at the opening of this chapter notes that "[Chiropractic] is carried on almost exclusively by those of no education, ignorant of anatomy, ignorant even of the fundamental sciences on which the treatment of disease depends." This editorial introduces a reprint of the statement of a Canton, Ohio judge as he imposed a $200 fine and 60 days in the workhouse on a chiropractor convicted of practicing medicine without a license. Included in the reprinted judge's comments is the following statement:

> For a long time there has been running in the magazines an advertisement: "Be a Doctor of Chiropractic, the new Drugless Healing Science of Spinal Adjustment; *a common school education is all you need to begin*; our simplified training does the rest." Men who believe in education, who glory in our school system, in our colleges, are staggered at his audaciousness.[30] (emphasis in the original)

The focus on the inadequate preparation of chiropractors intensifies after 1915 and continues through to the present time.

Between 1912 and 1923 there are five reports in JAMA of inspections of chiropractic colleges by orthodox physicians. These reports document the inadequate facilities, faculties, and curricula of the schools.[31] During this period there are two reports which document the lack of entrance requirements for students by publishing letters exchanged between stooge potential applicants to chiropractic schools and the admissions staff of these schools.[32] There are other items published throughout this early period, particularly during the second half of this period, which also focus on the lack of educational qualifications of chiropractors. These articles bemoan various aspects of chiropractic education including: mail-order plan or home study courses;[33] the little regard chiropractors have for education in general;[34] B.J. Palmer's statement that the Palmer School is established on a "Business not professional basis;"[35] the curriculum which includes salesmanship, "venomous propaganda" about the medical profession, and political organization;[36] and the flexibility of the so-called "requirement" of high school education by California chiropractic schools.[37] In each of these commentaries, chiropractic is denigrated.

Concern with the poor educational preparation of chiropractors is a theme which runs through NEJM at this point in history as well. Starting with the very first chiropractic-related item published in NEJM, the 1915 report of the conviction of a chiropractor for practicing medicine without a license, the judicial opinion regarding the power of the state to protect the public from ill-prepared practitioners is reprinted.[38] Throughout this early period chiropractors are referred to as "uneducated"[39] and "unqualified."[40] A reprint from the New York *Tribune* call chiropractors "innocent of medical knowledge" and asks "Why are they unwilling to come in [to medical practice] by the front door? Because they will not take the trouble to provide themselves with the key."[41] Some reports provide specifics on the inadequacy of chiropractic education, such as the 1923 report from St. Louis that a chiropractic degree was received after three evenings of study.[42]

Articles in NEJM cite the lack of adequate medical education as the primary reason for opposing legislation that would legalize the practice of chiropractic in Massachusetts by creating a separate Board of Chiropractic Examiners. Any efforts to create a separate board for chiropractors is seen as a lowering of standards.[43] Various editorials very explicitly state that opposition to chiropractic is not based on criticism of manipulation per se, but is rather based on the objection that it is performed by medically untrained practitioners. For example, a 1924 editorial states: "Physicians are not trying to interfere with the application of chiropractic methods if used by properly qualified doctors but are simply urging the state to maintain minimum educational standards for the benefit of the people."[44] In other items, of course, there *is* specific criticism of chiropractic treatment and the assumption appears to be that once the chiropractor receives proper medical training he will be, as Dr. Frothingham reported to the Suffolk District Medical Society in 1921, "an educated man and he will not practice chiropractic."[45]

Public Unable to Judge Chiropractic The concern over the lack of qualifications of chiropractors appears to be linked to a concern for public welfare since the assumption is that the general public is not qualified to judge the qualifications of health practitioners. For example, the previously noted reprint of a 1908 Oklahoma newspaper editorial states: "It is easy enough to mislead those who have absolutely no knowledge of medicine or anatomy...."[46] Similar sentiments are expressed throughout this period.[47] While at the beginning of this period JAMA appears to take a "hands off" or passive stance vis-a-vis this problem, this position soon switches to one recognizing a need for the protection of the public from chiropractic. For example, the 1908 reprinted newspaper editorial noted above concludes by saying "If a person is willing to place himself in the hands of such practitioners then it is none of our concern if the undertaker gets him."[48] A few years later, however, there are references to the importance of the medical practice acts in protecting the public from chiropractors.[49] Additionally, by the end of this period there are references to educating the public to the fallacy and hazards of chiropractic treatment. For example, in 1921 JAMA reprints an address by the Secretary of the Board of Medical Examiners in California wherein the question "Will an aggressive campaign of prosecution gradually drive out the violators by either forcing compliance with the law or, by means of some penalty imposed, drive the violator from the state?" is answered in the negative. Instead the speaker calls for a "campaign of education" to "convince the public that an individual untrained in the diagnosis of communicable disease is a serious public menace."[50]

The inability of the public to evaluate chiropractic is a theme woven throughout many of the NEJM items as well. It is frequently noted that the public is easily swayed by "sentiment" and does not realize the tremendous accomplishments of scientific medicine that are ignored by the chiropractors.[51] In contrast it is supposed that "intelligent citizens should quickly see through the fallacious propositions of the chiropractors."[52]

Information Updates In JAMA, very short informational updates that simply present information on current legislation regarding chiropractic practice acts are interspersed throughout the publication. Some of these are news items, some are in the "Medicolegal" section documenting cases where medical practice acts favoring orthodox practitioners are upheld, and some involve commentary on legislation.[53] These items do not specifically refer to the importance of legislation for consumer protection, but do point to the monitoring by the AMA of the legal status of chiropractic in the various states. While most of these items are implicitly negative, the information is presented in a more neutral and objective form.

The NEJM also includes this type of information update about chiropractic, primarily focusing on the legislation that is being considered in Massachusetts. But there are also articles that provide informational updates on chiropractic legislation in other states, such as the big conflicts in New York and California that were the focus of attention in JAMA as well.[54] There is particular interest in legislation in the New England states, most of which adopted laws allowing chiropractors to practice by 1921.[55]

Reference to Class Origins of Chiropractors There also appears to be some element of status or class conflict involved in medical references to chiropractic, with the view that these "common school educated" practitioners can not possibly have anything to offer to contemporary health care practices. The evidence of this view is usually quite subtle during the first part of this period as illustrated in the quote with which this chapter begins, referring to chiropractic as a "trade" not a profession and to the "audaciousness" of chiropractic claims.[56] More explicit illustrations of this conflict appear more frequently during the latter part of this period. For example, in 1916 JAMA editors refer to chiropractic as "an illegitimate offspring of a plebeian cult of aristocratic aspirations."[57] Other items refer to the previous occupations of chiropractors, which are typically low status occupations. A Pennsylvania physician writes to JAMA saying:

> On the day I left my home and office in July, 1917, for the Army this man, who is now a "chiropractor," was perched on a ladder across the street painting a house. Six months later in camp, I received my home newspaper containing his noisy advertisement. He had acquired the prefix "Dr." and was flourishing.[58]

The editorial commentary accompanying this letter continues:

> It is ... inconceivable that a man with a few weeks' reading of law would be admitted to the bar and entrusted with cases that might involve large financial interests. But a street cleaner or garbage collector can take a six months' "course" in "chiropractic" and be permitted by the commonwealth to hold himself out as competent to treat the most complicated piece of mechanism known - the human body.[59]

Other items refer to the previous occupations of chiropractors as ditch-diggers,[60] and "ignorant mechanics, clerks, and even ne'er-do-wells."[61] A 1924 commentary refers to the Universal Chiropractors Association as the "Amalgamated Order of Spine-Pushers."[62] These references to the working-class or lower-class origins of chiropractors reveal an element of class or status conflict between orthodox physicians and chiropractors that goes beyond the rejection of chiropractors on scientific or educational grounds alone.

Similarly, in a column entitled "Confessions of a Chiropractor," a Utah advertisement is quoted to show how little regard chiropractors have for education. The advertisement is quoted as saying that Greek and Latin are "Both dead tongues and, outside those engaged in translating manuscripts, are used only to display pedantry; they are of no value to chiropractors." [63] The column goes on to discuss chiropractors' disdain for the study of bacteriology, chemistry, and other aspects of *materia medica*. But the particular quote reprinted above reveals the class distinctions that are being drawn between the physician and the chiropractor The classical education model, which was certainly the model for the education of the upper classes, is being rejected by the chiropractor who is quoted, thereby confirming his lower-class standing. It is very interesting that the chiropractor is knowingly placing himself below the perceived higher social class standing of the physician, perhaps emphasizing his similarity to his clientele.

There are fewer such direct references to the lower class origins of chiropractors in the pages of NEJM, although the 1921 report by Dr. Frothingham does mention that chiropractic was started by a layman, "rumor has it by a man who drove the buggy for a successful osteopath."[64] However, recognition of the social class differences between physicians and chiropractors -- and the role this plays in the conflict between chiropractors and physicians -- is evident in more subtle ways. There are two areas in which the concern with social class is evident in NEJM. One is the debate over the appropriate strategy for orthodox medicine to adopt in regard to chiropractic and other cults. The second is the criticism of the tactics used by chiropractors in their push for legislative reform.

The debate over the type of strategy that should be used in opposing chiropractic in Massachusetts basically assumes the following form. On the one hand there are those who argue with upper class assurance that right is on their side, that chiropractic and the other cults will naturally disappear and that if physicians criticize chiropractic it will appear as if it is worthy of physician attention, which it is not. It is considered to be beneath the dignity of the medical profession to engage in such efforts. On the other hand, there are those who argue that physicians must take an active stance in fighting chiropractic and the other cults, for right cannot win without assistance. In 1921 an editorial warns[65] "If we sit with folded hands, or as pacifists, we must not later deplore a situation to which neglect may have contributed some support." Likewise, a 1924 editorial says:

> The weakness of medical men in arguments employed to influence the people has seemed to lie in the dignity and conservatism of well-equipped physicians. The advocates of chiropractic have not been accused of modesty.[66]

When the chiropractic bills are defeated later in the decade, particular mention is made of the fact that all actions by physicians in the campaign were dignified.[67]

UNITY, STATUS, DOMINANCE AND OUTRAGE AT CHIROPRACTIC

We now turn to the central issue in this chapter: how the medical profession's reaction of incredulity and outrage at chiropractic is part of the changes that are taking place in medicine as it strives to become a unified profession of high social status that dominates the health care arena.

The Development of Medical Unity

There are two major developments taking place at the beginning of this century that are part of the effort to generate medical unity. First, the AMA launches a major campaign to unify the profession organizationally. Second, the profession is clearly trying to develop a unified image and identity. Each of these developments -- and how the medical reaction to chiropractic is part of these developments -- will be discussed below.

Organizational Unity As I note in chapter 2 regarding the history of medicine, a major reorganization of the AMA and its relations with state and local medical societies takes place in 1901. Up until that point, membership in the association is not open to all physicians; rather, membership consists of delegates from the state medical societies and those members who are admitted "by application." In the new federalized scheme of organization, general membership in the AMA is integrated with membership in local and state medical societies. Local medical societies elect delegates to the state medical societies which in turn elect delegates to sit in the House of Delegates of the AMA, a central part of the governance structure of the association.

The new organizational form for the AMA is the result of many factors, of course, but primary among these is the perception that the orthodox medical profession needs greater unification. The cry for greater unity in the medical profession is issued in numerous editorials in JAMA at the turn of the century. Unity is defined more broadly than a concern with AMA reorganization, however. The following excerpt from an 1896 editorial, for example, decries the lack of unity within the profession and links this lack of unity to the low esteem of the medical profession and the use of "quacks" by the public.

> The esteem of the public for the profession may be most aptly synonymized by the word disesteem. And this disesteem is very largely due to the fact that the profession has heretofore shown little or no *esprit de corps*, and has been inexcusably weak in permitting the contempt of the world to stand as a confession of just judgment.... The evils of quackery exist because we are

not united in crushing them out of existence, and in the estimation of the public our failure to do this is due to the fact that we are half-quacks ourselves, with but a faint-hearted belief in the therapeutic value or scientific quality of our own "science". It is one of the strangest facts of modern sociology that so large a body of men as we have no professional unity, that we present no united front to the enemies of our guild or to the public influences prejudicial to public health. Every other calling or occupation bands itself together and seeks to influence legislation or popular feeling by a hundred instrumentalities while we are content not only to do little or nothing and what little we do sporadically and by individual imitation and energy, but we allow our thousand enemies to deride us and "walk over us" by their unanimous and organized opposition.[68]

Published in 1896, only one year after chiropractic begins, this editorial is not written in response to any particular challenge by chiropractic. Yet it indicates just how the need for unity was conceptualized by leaders in JAMA: as a tool that once secured could be used both to increase the prestige of the profession in the eyes of the public and to eliminate the "enemies of our guild" and the "public influences prejudicial to public health."

There are numerous editorials around the turn of the century that express similar ideas regarding the need for unity and the benefits of such for both the profession and the public. The message is clear: unity would allow the profession to effectively oppose certain groups and activities and to promote others. This link between the call for unity and the elimination of "quackery" is central to this analysis. Therefore I will provide several examples of editorials in which this link appears.

Another 1896 editorial, entitled "The Power and Force of a United Profession," begins with the flattering but perhaps inaccurate assertion that

Every intelligent and reflecting physician must recognize the power and force of the medical profession of this country when united in an effort to accomplish such legislation as may be deemed conducive to public welfare and to the advancement of scientific medicine.[69]

But the editorial, which deals with proposed anti-vivisection legislation, then goes on to exhort:

Will the profession wait until the crisis comes? Will it rest supinely in fancied security until defeat and disaster are impending, or will it assert the prerogatives of scientific medicine, and by united effort enforce them in the interest of, and for the welfare of mankind, in that governors, legislative bodies, town councils and all others in authority may come to know that in preventive and remedial medicine *truth and science must dominate fanaticism, whim, caprice, charlatanry and mercenary adventure.*[70] (emphasis added)

A lengthy abstract of an article pleading for unification of the medical profession (more than twice as long as the typical review) is included in an 1899 review of "Current Medical Literature." The review reads in part:

> We ignore the truth that in union there is strength and subdivide our efforts and waste our energies. There are in the United States nearly one hundred thousand members of the regular profession. Imagine our power socially and practically if we paid allegiance to one national association, for instance, the one that has always taken the lead in power and numbers, viz., the American Medical Association. This should be strengthened by an enormously increased membership to which every physician should feel the same loyalty as to the country in which he lives.[71]

An 1899 editorial praises an attempt in England to establish a national medical guild that will focus on "medicopolitical rather than scientific" objectives and calls for some type of such organization in the United States saying:

> *What with ... charlatanry of every stripe in every part of the country, there is certainly need of an organization on the part of the medical profession.* Aside from any commercial or professional reason, our duty to our patients justifies organized effort on the part of the medical profession for the purpose of eliminating these hordes which seem to be springing up more than ever and in various disguises.... The remedy for existing evils lies in enforcement of state laws and enactment of new ones if necessary. In the few instances in which the physicians of a state have thoroughly organized, satisfactory results have always been accomplished. A united profession in any state is a political power which is always respected, and its desires are generally granted.[72] (emphasis added)

This editorial clearly illustrates how unity of the profession is seen as a necessary precursor for the effective pursuit of medicine's interests, which are again depicted in this case as the advancement of science for the welfare of humankind. It also illustrates again the link between unity and the reaction against "quackery".

An editorial in 1900 praises the efforts of Iowa physicians to prevent the Congressional nomination of a state senator who had supported osteopathy in an earlier legislative battle. The editorial concludes:

When legislators are made to recognize the influence of the medical profession unselfishly exhorted in favor of right objects they will be *less ready to follow the dictation of quacks* than they seem too often to be at present. That influence can be exercised when the profession is organized.[73] (emphasis added)

A 1901 editorial in the "Minor Comment" section of JAMA warns members of the medical profession to follow the activities of their state legislatures. Citing a proposed amendment to the Illinois medical practice act which would exempt those who treat the sick by massage or spiritual means as the kind of legislation that can slip past an unwary profession, the editor chastises: "When this occurs, nine times out of ten it is the fault of the profession itself, a result of lack of organization and of apathy."[74]

These examples, which come from editorials that deal with a variety of topics, clearly reveal the ways in which the cry for unity is so frequently related to the call to eliminate charlatanry.

The reorganization of the AMA in 1901 contributes to the unification of the profession, but is more a beginning point for unification than an end point. Recognizing this, the AMA hires Dr. Joseph McCormack as a field organizer. Between 1900 and 1911 McCormack travels all over the U.S. addressing medical and lay audiences. Burrow (1977) says there were three major goals of this organizational crusade: 1) to organize medical societies in areas where there were none and to revitalize those which were inactive; 2) to promote professional unity; and 3) to establish a positive image of the profession.

By most accounts, McCormack's efforts are a success. In 1901, the AMA has 10,600 members; by 1906, it has 60,000 members (Fishbein 1947, pp. 203, 216). But significant as the almost six-fold increase in AMA membership is, it would be a mistake to assume that the medical profession has achieved "unity" by 1906. The reorganized and larger AMA has perhaps greater diversity among its membership than ever before.

Unified Collective Identity At the turn of the century and into the first decades of this century the orthodox medical profession is composed of physicians with different and sometimes competing interests: specialists versus generalists; those supporting proprietary interests versus those supporting non-proprietary organizations; those in hospital and dispensary practice versus those in private practice; those supporting the advertisement of services versus those opposing such advertisement; medical school faculty versus medical practitioners; and so on. Throughout the early part of this century, the orthodox medical profession was very much involved in defining itself as a profession and defining exactly what that meant. Looking at the above controversies, it is clear that many of these issues are identity or definitional controversies as well as economic conflicts. For example, in the debate over advertisement (which was prohibited by the AMA Code of Ethics) there is, of course, an economic issue at stake. Advertising -- either of rates or skills -- could potentially give certain practitioners a competitive edge. But there is also a definitional issue at stake. Advertising is a tool of the patent medicine hawker, the sectarians, and (as the orthodox practitioners defined them) the quacks. Do the regular physicians want to use tactics that were associated with these unsavory groups? Leaders of the major medical organizations, such as the AMA, answer that question in the negative. As will be discussed in the next section, these leaders want to secure the identity of "profession" not "trade" for the orthodox practitioners and in their view, that excludes advertising.

The controversy over proprietary medical schools is another example where unity of image and identity is involved. This controversy is in part a quality-of-medical-education issue, since the proprietary schools typically offer a poorer quality of education than the nonproprietary institutions. It is in part an economic issue, since the large number of proprietary school graduates are blamed for the oversupply of physicians (which are in turn seen as responsible for a decline in physician incomes). But this controversy is also in part an image and identity issue. For example, in a 1912 JAMA article Gordon Rice, M.D. writes:

> [H]ow many [people] would know the difference between the work done in the best, fully equipped medical school and that done in the half-baked business institution that turns out raw and ignorant practitioners for the profit received from fees? ... We have at least three grades of legalized medical schools, classed as A, B and C by the Committee on Medical Education of the American Medical Association, and the product of the poorest is equal, in the eyes of the law and of the public, to that of the best. The public dubs a man "doctor" whether his training was an eight weeks' "optometry" course, a correspondence course from a "mechano-therapy" or "chiropractic" institution, a nine-months course in neurology or the course required by the best university in the land.[75]

This quotation illustrates how the question of proprietary medical schools is in part an issue of the image and collective identity of the medical profession being developed at this point in history. The proprietary medical schools typically provide a low quality education that is not in keeping with the professional identity and image being promoted by the AMA. Proprietary schools are associated with the sectarian or irregular schools and the orthodox medical profession is distancing itself from these irregulars. A

1914 editorial in JAMA contrasts chiropractic and orthodox medical education:

> The so called "colleges" of chiropractic matriculate anybody who can pay the fee. The medical school requires, in addition to a good preliminary educational foundation, four years -- in some cases five -- of hard study with much practical work before granting the degree of doctor of medicine.[76]

In reading this, it is important to remember that although medical school education had generally begun to improve during the preceding twenty years, the "pay-the-fee" requirement existed in some medical schools until only a few years before this editorial is written .

Conclusion I have argued that the unity sought by the leaders of the medical profession -- organizationally and in terms of collective identity and image -- was generated by the opposition to irregular practitioners, including chiropractors. That is, in the process of opposing the irregular practitioners the orthodox medical profession established a collective identity, a collective image, a unity of purpose and a unified professional association.

I am not suggesting that the orthodox medical profession intentionally opposed chiropractic and other sectarians because they needed to achieve unity. I am suggesting instead that the leaders of the medical profession perceived a need to increase the unity among members of the profession and that one of the primary means of accomplishing this was through the opposition to the irregulars, including chiropractic. I see no evidence of a conscious, intentional effort to target the irregular practitioners in order to achieve this unity. But there is much evidence, as I have shown, that the movement to increase unity -- both organizationally and in terms of collective identity and image -- is consistently linked to opposition to these practitioners. The plea for a unified professional association is couched in terms of successfully fighting the quacks and charlatans. The efforts to construct a collective identity and image are couched in terms of differentiating the orthodox profession from the irregular practitioners.

Securing a Favorable Social Position

In the previous section I discussed how orthodox medicine was involved in a quest for unity of image and identity at the turn of the century and the first few decades of this century. In discussing this quest, I noted that there were many competing interests within the orthodox profession and very different ideas about the appropriate organization of medical practice (which would reflect a particular professional identity and image). In that section I focused upon the process of achieving unity and how medical reactions to chiropractic and other sectarians were an integral part of the process. In this section I want to focus more on the substance of this process. The basic point here is that while orthodox practitioners increased their unity through the process of establishing image and collective identity, the particular image and identity they sought to develop (one of high class, status and power) was linked to the concrete effort to improve the collective social position of physicians in this country.

The social position of the orthodox physician at the turn of the century is not as clearly prestigious or economically secure as it is today. While there is some disagreement over the social position of physicians at this time,[77] most JAMA publications are similar to the 1896 editorial quoted earlier that clearly decries the "disesteem" in which physicians are held. The need for increased prestige is one that is acknowledged repeatedly. It is something that the profession appears to see as well-deserved. In an 1896 editorial entitled "Lay Distrust and Enmity of the Medical Profession," for example, the author bemoans the suspicions and opposition of the laity to the medical profession as indicated by their failure to provide financial support for medical education, opposition to vaccinations, continued support of the patent medicine industry and the general hatred and "bitterness of spirit against physicians" that is exhibited in some popular media (such as cartoons protesting vivisection).[78] This lack of esteem for the profession is tied back to the lack of unity in the profession by a physician reader who responds to this editorial. "The trouble," he says, "lies within our own circle...,"[79] referring to the ways in which physicians publicly criticize colleagues, giving a bad impression to laity.

An 1897 editorial refers to the low social esteem of physicians and links this to the over-supply of physicians.

> [T]he public estimation of the profession appears to have, in a measure, grown in an inverse ratio to its increase in numbers. We have cheapened ourselves by making ourselves too common.

> The medical profession is said to have led all the other so-called learned professions last year in the number of suicides of its members, a not very enviable distinction, but one that it may continue to hold if its numbers continue to increase with a correspondingly cheapened popular estimation.[80]

Another illustration of the issue of social status (and economic status) arises in a somewhat oblique editorial regarding "acrimonious exchanges" at a meeting of the AMA. One of the issues under discussion at the meeting and in the editorial was the issue of the Code of Ethics, in particular its prohibition of advertising.

> We can but conclude that it is hardly the Code which is at the bottom of the "hard times" but over-production and over-inducements. As a profession, at least those who are stranded in it have only the redress of restricted immigration since with all the minute division into specialties and the fads of multi-millionaires, we can not expect much gratitude and still less recognition. The no-coders say in effect: "It is the public's right and the world owes every man a living; so let none of us withdraw our small talents from the field, but incontinently convert our profession into a trade. We may then peddle our wares from door to door, and perhaps earn a mansion - in the skies."[81]

This editorial reveals a number of concerns of the orthodox profession that are relevant to the issues being considered here. It reveals again the concern with the social position of the profession as a whole. It demonstrates the debate over the appropriate path for medicine to follow (stop advertising? reduce supply of physicians?). It illustrates the views held by the leaders of the AMA and shows how these views are linked to social and economic status concerns. The editorial argues that it is better to be a profession than a trade; if particular physicians want to advertise, it may help them earn a living, but the collective social and economic status of the profession will suffer.

Conclusion The concern regarding the status of the profession is linked to the reaction to chiropractic as outrage during this period. As discussed earlier in this chapter, the orthodox medical profession frequently juxtaposed themselves with the chiropractors and other sectarian practitioners in the process of developing a collective image and identity: They advertise; we do not. They have poor training and preparation; we have rigorous training. They are a trade; we are a profession. As you will recall from earlier in this chapter, there were frequent references in the pages of JAMA to the lower-class status of chiropractors: to their previous occupations as ditch-diggers, fish-mongers and house painters; to their "noisy" advertisements; to their common school education and disdain for the university training of physicians.

The outrage against chiropractic can be viewed two ways. First, the outrage can be viewed as basically a dependent phenomenon. Just as the orthodox profession is working to establish a favorable social position for itself, along come the chiropractors with their relatively low social class standing, claiming to offer treatment for all diseases and rejecting the superiority of orthodox medicine and orthodox physicians. The outrage is a reaction to what chiropractors are doing. But the outrage must also be analyzed from another point of view, which looks at how the very process of securing a favorable social status for itself involves demonstrating the low social status of chiropractors. This view recognizes the outrage expressed toward chiropractic as an integral part of orthodox practitioners' own efforts to increase their social and economic status. It is *through* the denunciation of the inferiority of chiropractic that orthodox medicine affirms its superiority.

Securing Dominance

The third significant set of changes taking place after the turn of the century is the effort to secure a dominant position for orthodox physicians with respect to other healing practitioners and an autonomous position with respect to the State.[82] These efforts were clearly related to the call for medical unity and the efforts to increase the status of medicine discussed above and to the opposition of orthodox medicine to chiropractic at this point in history. I again ask you to recall the circumstances of medicine at the turn of the century. Orthodox medicine has not yet solidified its domination in the medical arena. It is in the process of doing so. Orthodox physicians are not yet seen as providing services that are clearly superior to those that can be provided by the untrained or by those trained in other healing sects.

In a turn-of-the-century editorial entitled "Medical Makeshifts" the editor decries the makeshift manner in which medical matters are handled by local and federal administrators and urges physicians to push for change. The article expresses outrage over the tale told by an ex-Army cavalry officer who had recently ended duty at an Army Recruiting Rendezvous. This officer reported that he had never worked with a medical examiner but had conducted the physical examination of recruits himself. The editorial responds to this report saying:

> Nothing can justify the makeshift principle which requires an incompetent individual to discharge duties for which a sufficient number of qualified officers ought to be provided.... Whether it be two hundred or three hundred or more thoroughly qualified medical officers who are required for the proper performance of these duties, they should be obtained at whatever cost, and no pretense of economy can ever justify their substitution in a single instance or under any circumstances, by incompetent makeshifts.[83]

This editorial provides a good example of how orthodox physicians are trying to secure occupational task boundaries and establish their dominance in the medical arena. The editorial strenuously objects to nonphysicians performing what they claim to be "their work." This example is particularly interesting because today, in the 1990s, it is not at all uncommon for a nonphysician such as a nurse practitioner or physician assistant to conduct routine physical examinations. The difference, of course, is that today these nonphysicians perform under the direction and authority of physicians. At the turn of the century physicians had not yet secured the dominant position in the medical arena and did not yet have the authority to control the practice of medicine. Nonphysicians performed physical examinations because the idea that such exams were in the physician's domain did not exist; the "physician's domain" did not exist.

But organized medicine was working toward securing this domain and the editorial quoted above is one example of these efforts. There are many examples of this push for medical dominance. Editorials bemoan the influence of nonphysicians in medical affairs and argue that physicians must have authority over medical matters. A 1900 editorial states:

> While, then, strictly speaking, the medical man may not be able to devote himself to matters of finance and business with the same force as his lay colleague, *he must yet be recognized as an authority at least on medical matters* whether in the direction of education or of hospital organization and management. The plan, therefore, seems a wise one, to retain on boards of trustees of medical colleges and hospitals several physicians ... who can be trusted to serve with distinction and usefulness *in places that can not be filled by any other than physicians*.[84] (emphasis added)

Again, this editorial illustrates the efforts of AMA leaders to push the claim that orthodox physicians should have exclusive authority over matters medical and to secure dominance in these areas.

The efforts to secure dominance and autonomy are most clearly seen in the legal battles over the licensing of medical practice. As you will recall from chapter 2, the seat of authority for medical licensing has shifted historically. According to Shyrock (1967), licensing was handled through the medical schools from 1839 to 1875. After 1875 the medical societies became interested once again in the licensing issue (as they had been prior to 1830) and in fact attempted to improve the quality of medical school education by promoting licensing by state boards (also popular before 1830). Shyrock (1967, p. 112) notes that "this process, although a gradual one until 1900, proceeded rapidly during the next two decades," which are the decades of interest here.

What is important, as far as the discussion here is concerned, is that legal regulation of orthodox medicine is very closely linked to the legal regulation of other forms of medical practice as well. That is, the very consideration of orthodox medicine's own regulation involves consideration of the regulation of "quackery." My argument here is the same as that in the preceding two sections: just as opposition to quackery in general and chiropractic in particular is part of the very process by which orthodox medicine sought unity and an increase in status, this opposition is integral to efforts to establish medical dominance, including legal domination.

An 1896 editorial illustrates the renewed concern with the regulation of medicine at the turn of the century and is an example of how the "quackery" issue is central to this discussion.

It is high time that the American medical profession should ask the American people if it is the proper function of our Government to enact and execute laws furthering the science of medicine and therefore the health of the community and the progress of civilization, or whether it is much longer to ignore these noble purposes and continue to support downright quackery?[85]

Medical practice laws, then as now, specify the activities in which the various healing practitioners may engage and, through the establishment of various boards and examination procedures, specify who qualifies as particular types of practitioners. It is here at this basic legal level that status and dominance were secured for it is the medical practice laws that specified that certain activities, such as surgery and the prescription of medications, could only be performed by physicians. The medical practice laws that were passed at the beginning of this century very clearly placed physicians at the top of the medical hierarchy and others, such as pharmacists, below them. But more fundamentally, these laws also created a new sphere of acceptable and legal medical practice and practitioners that excluded other existing health practitioners.

The orthodox medical opposition to chiropractic was central in these battles over the legal regulation of medicine. As you will recall from the beginning of this chapter, all of the items published in JAMA regarding chiropractic during the early part of the first period (1908 to 1911) concern the legal regulation of chiropractic and the prosecution of chiropractors for practicing medicine without a license. This topic continues to be a dominant theme throughout the rest of the early period as well, with 51 of the total of 104 items published in JAMA from 1912 to 1924 related to the legal regulation of chiropractic in some fashion.[86] This demonstrates the centrality of regulation issues to orthodox organized medicine's interest in chiropractic.

But in order to make the point that orthodox medical opposition to chiropractic was central to its own efforts to secure dominance it is necessary to examine other evidence from this period. One such piece of evidence is a 1921 JAMA editorial titled "A Service Rendered by Chiropractors." This editorial concludes that chiropractors are performing a service by forcing the courts to address the constitutionality of state medical practice laws.

> Good frequently results from opposition and it seems that actual benefit may result from the attacks on scientific medical practice made by chiropractors in their attempts to secure exemption from medical practice laws. Most states have excellent laws regarding the practice of medicine, but the constitutionality of many of these laws has not been tested in the courts. Thanks to the chiropractors, not only are these tests being applied, but the decisions rendered are tending *to show more clearly what constitutes the practice of medicine....* Chiropractors have been unhindered in their practice for so long that they have come to consider themselves immune from medical practice laws.... Any law which restricts them, therefore, is declared to be "a discrimination," and on that claim they undertake to have the law declared unconstitutional. In fact, available evidence indicates a nationwide campaign to invalidate medical practice laws.... The tests should be applied also to the laws establishing separate boards for certain groups of practitioners and lower educational standards than are required of physicians. These laws are clearly class legislation and discriminate against physicians. Just as soon as the basic and essential needs are presented to the judiciary, an outcome favorable to education and common sense will be assured.[87] (emphasis added)

This editorial nicely illustrates how organized medicine's battle with chiropractic is integrally related to its efforts to outline its task boundaries and secure dominance over that domain.[88] This editorial is also interesting because it shows how JAMA leaders themselves construe a positive functionalist interpretation of their battle with chiropractic.

Organized medicine couched most of the discussion of the legal regulation of chiropractic in terms of the poor training of chiropractors. Orthodox medical practitioners saw their superior educational qualifications as justifying their dominant position in the medical arena. Their basic argument was that chiropractors were not sufficiently educated to treat the human body and they therefore should not be legally recognized at all or, as was frequently suggested in the second half of this early period, they should be required to have the same medical training as orthodox physicians. The latter is seen as an insurmountable block for chiropractors and therefore in effect no different from banning chiropractic practice.

By any standard of measure it is clear that orthodox medicine did require a higher level of preliminary and medical preparation. But just as I argued earlier that orthodox medicine's opposition to chiropractic and other healing sects was part of its own effort to seek unity and higher social status, so too do I argue that this opposition is part of its effort to secure medical dominance. Orthodox physicians do not merely oppose chiropractic because they reject the low educational standards of chiropractic; both the opposition to chiropractic and the rejection of the poor preparation of chiropractors are *part of* organized medicine's efforts to establish a dominant position in the medical arena. Organized medicine can publicize its own educational requirements as it denounces the lack of same among chiropractors.

The argument that legal recognition of chiropractic hinges on its educational preparation is given over and over again in this early period, particularly in the second half of the period. A 1915 editorial touts a Supreme Court decision (regarding osteopathy) saying:

In the treatment of human ailments the matter of primary importance to the conscientious practitioner is the diagnosis. What is causing the trouble? On the answer to this question depends the treatment, no matter whether the "doctor" is a physician, an osteopath, a chiropractor, a mental healer, or what not. The diagnosis is the essential and unless the "doctor" is sufficiently well trained to make a diagnosis, he is not qualified to treat the patient intelligently by any method whatever....

The court, therefore, decisively pushed aside the masses of argument regarding the "rights" of this, that or the other medical sect, and revealed the real point at issue - the necessity for sufficient fundamental knowledge of the human system to qualify one to make a diagnosis. The court emphasized that in order to make a diagnosis the practitioner of osteopathy, or any other cult, must have the same scientific training as is required of physicians. *It is clearly the duty of the state, therefore, to provide an educational qualification which will guarantee that every licensed practitioner shall be competent to make an intelligent diagnosis.* Certainly the public has a right to expect that only those who are competent will be given the state's endorsement, conferring on them the right to treat human ailments.[89] (emphasis added)

Duhigg's opening statement in his 1915 article "Where Chiropractors Are Made" provides another illustration of the concern of orthodox practitioners with the legalization of practice by poorly trained chiropractors. Duhigg takes his information from a report by the Inspector of the Pennsylvania Bureau of Medical Education and Licensure, who visited three chiropractic schools in Iowa.

As the season for legislation approaches, I feel that the information that I have concerning chiropractors should be put at the disposal of those interested in guarding the public health and maintaining respectable educational standards.... These reports set forth everything with painful exactness and embarrassing detail. Any patriotic legislator will be justly incensed at the thought of taking the intellectual refuse from these schools who are not licensed to practice in Iowa, to be used in his own state as the guardians of life and health. They should not be given legal recognition to practice in any state. If they are permitted to practice, it should be only after they have obtained the same professional and preliminary training that is required of physicians....[90]

This example not only shows the link between education and the legal regulation issue, but also provides an example of how the dominance of orthodox medicine is implied in the suggestion that chiropractors, if they are not banned totally, should be required to meet the same educational standards as those of orthodox medicine (the "highest" standards for the "highest" group). This quotation also captures the sense of outrage that typifies this first period.

A final example of the way in which orthodox medicine links its concern with the poor preparation of chiropractors to the legal regulation issue is provided in a 1923 column in JAMA's "The Propaganda for Reform" section entitled "The Menace of Chiropractic." In this column, the editor says that in contrast to the cult practitioners' assertion that medical practice legislation exists to protect physicians, such legislation clearly protects the public. Focusing on chiropractic, the editorial states:

> This cult menaces public health, not because its devotees advertise by circus-like methods, nor even because the theory on which it is based is the unscientific and preposterous one that all diseases are due to subluxated vertebrae impinging on spinal nerves. No, the chief reason is that those who call themselves chiropractors are uneducated men who know practically nothing of the human body and its intricate mechanism. Chiropractors are uneducated because the so-called chiropractic colleges are not educational institutions but "trade schools" which cater to the ignorant and the venal....[91]

The column continues with a comparison of the low standards for entrance to chiropractic school with the high standards for entrance to medical school. Again, this quotation provides an illustration of how organized medicine couches its interest in the legal regulation of chiropractic in terms of its concern with the poor preparation of chiropractors and how in doing so it announces its own high standards which justify a dominant position in the medical arena. The quotation also captures the sense of outrage expressed so often in this first period.

Conclusion: Unity, Status, Dominance and Outrage at Chiropractic

I characterized the early medical literature regarding chiropractic in terms of "outrage." Placed in the historical context of the push for unity, status, and dominance, this view of chiropractic as an outrage -- as opposed to some other negative reaction -- is quite understandable. After all, since the mid-1890s the medical profession had been struggling mightily to upgrade itself -- to increase the quality of education, to increase the status and income of practitioners, to improve the collective image of the profession, and to secure its dominant position in the field of medicine. By 1910, when the medical profession finally begins to take notice of chiropractic, they consider themselves well into the final stages of "cleaning their own house" and on the verge of assuming their deserved dominant position in society in general and the medical world in particular. Then along comes chiropractic, refusing to disappear (as did most of the other irregular practices). Not only does chiropractic not disappear but it appears to grow rapidly. When news comes that the Palmer School of Chiropractic has over two thousand students enrolled in 1921, the reaction is swift. Chiropractic might have been treated as too absurd to consider in 1910, but a few years later -- and clearly in 1921 -- the reaction expressed is outrage.

Outrage is a fitting reaction; the outrage reaction is one of "How dare they?!" It is the reaction of a group that perceives itself as superior to a group it perceives as inferior. It is a reaction of the dominant to the subordinate.[92] In these early years of the century, the orthodox medical profession is striving for and establishing its dominance. Expressing outrage is one way of both affirming and creating that dominance.

NOTES

1. From the "Current Comment" section of JAMA, July 26, 1913, 61(4): 284-5.
2. The first entries regarding chiropractic are:
     JAMA May 23, 1908, 50(21):1697 (one sentence in "Medical News" section under "Iowa");
     JAMA May 23, 1908, 50(21):1715 (five sentences in "Medical Economics" section plus a reprint of an editorial from the Oklahoma City *Times* which credits physicians in the state senate with the defeat of this bill);
     JAMA June 20, 1908, 50(25):2077 (one sentence in the "Medical Economics" section).
3. These items are, respectively:
     JAMA Mar. 20, 1909, 52(12):981 (in "Medical Economics" section);
     JAMA Mar. 27, 1909, 52(13):1048 (in "Medical News - New York");

JAMA Sept. 18, 1909, 53(12):958 (in "Medical News - Washington").

4.   JAMA Feb. 19, 1910, 54(8):621 (in "Medical News - Missouri"). Other JAMA items mentioning chiropractic in 1910 are :

JAMA May 28, 1910, 54(22):1794 (in "Medical News - Iowa");

JAMA June 11, 1910, 54(24):1970, 1972 (two separate items in "Minutes of the House of Delegates");

JAMA Dec. 10, 1920, 55(24):2070 (in "Medical News - Illinois").

5.   These four entries are in the following JAMA issues, respectively:

July 29, 1911, 57(5):412-413;

Aug. 5, 1911, 57(6):501;

Sept. 9, 1911, 57(11):924;

Nov. 25, 1911, 57(22):1795.

6.   JAMA May 23, 1908, 50(21):1715.

7.   Gordon W. Rice, M.D., "Pseudoscience," JAMA Feb.3, 1912, 58(5):360-362.

8.   For examples, see the following JAMA issues:

July 26, 1913, 61(4):284-5;

Aug. 26, 1916, 67(9):686 (quotes advertisement concerning infantile paralysis);

March 3, 1917, 68(9):732 (reprint of explanation of governor of Hawaii for vetoing chiropractic bill);

Nov. 23, 1918, 71(21):1764 (pictured advertisement for using chiropractic to fight flu);

July 19, 1919, 73(3):213 (copy of letter encouraging someone to seek chiropractic care);

May 15, 1920, 74(20):1407 (reprint of N.J. definition of chiropractic);

Oct. 30, 1920, 75(18):1209 (quotes chiropractic advertisement on cause of gall stones);

Nov. 6, 1920, 75 (19):1276 (quotes B.J. Palmer on his chiropractic school being established on a business not professional basis).

9.   BMSJ Dec. 29, 1921, 185(26):799.

10. BMSJ Nov. 8, 1923, 189(19):717.

11. BMSJ Dec. 29, 1921, 185(26):799.

12. BMSJ Apr. 3, 1924, 190(14):610.

13. JAMA Aug. 23, 1919, 73(8):615.

14. JAMA May 15, 1920, 74(20):1407.

15. JAMA Feb. 5, 1921, 76(6):385.

16. JAMA Feb. 5, 1921, 76(6):385.

17. JAMA July 16, 1921, 77(3):220.

18. JAMA Sept. 17, 1921, 77(12):944.

19. JAMA Oct. 1, 1921, 77(19):1122.

20. JAMA July 26, 1913, 61(4):284; JAMA Apr. 11, 1914, 62(15):1177.

21. JAMA Mar. 10, 1923, 80(10):715.

22. *Ibid.*

23. JAMA Nov. 3, 1923, 81(18):1493.

24. As noted elsewhere, most of the chiropractic-related publications in BMSJ/NEJM appear in the 1920s and 1930s. The editorial staff of NEJM seem to have distances themselves from the chiropractic issue, although I can find no report of such an

editorial policy. The peak years for articles concerning chiropractic are 1927, 1931 and 1932, which puts the peak for NEJM a few years later for NEJM than JAMA. This relates to the appearance of chiropractic bills before the Massachusetts legislature during the late twenties and early thirties, since NEJM is the journal of the Massachusetts Medical Society.

25. BMSJ May 8, 1924, 190(19):811.

26. NEJM Apr. 9, 1931, 204(15):782-783.

27. NEJM Feb. 11, 1932, 206(6):299.

28. BMSJ Oct. 25, 1923, 189(17):626. This is a copy of a letter sent to the Veterans' Bureau by the secretary of the Massachusetts Medical Society to discourage the use of chiropractic treatment in the Veterans' Bureau.

29. BMSJ May 5, 1927, 196(18):750. This comes from an article in the *Texas State Journal of Medicine* (April 1927) that a reader sent to BMSJ because "I thought it might be of interest in your fight against chiropractic."

30. JAMA July 26, 1913, 61(4):284-5 (appears in "Current Comment").

31. These five reports are:

    1)   Thomas F. Duhigg, M.D., "Where Chiropractors Are Made," JAMA Dec. 25, 1915, 65(26):2228-2229 (an article reporting visits to three chiropractic schools in Iowa, in which chiropractic students are referred to as "intellectual refuse");

    2)   "A Chiropractic Doctor Factory," JAMA Mar. 24, 1917, 68(12):932 (a report in the "Medical Education and State Boards of Registration" section);

    3)   "The Fountainhead of Chiropractic; What of Its Product?" JAMA July 13, 1920, 75(1):52-53 (a report in the "Medical Education, Registration, and Hospital Service" section);

    4)   George Dock, M.D., "A Visit to a Chiropractic School," JAMA Jan. 7, 1922, 78(1):60-63 (a report of a visit to Palmer School of Chiropractic in the section "Medical Education, Registration and Hospital Service section);

    5)   "More Diploma Mills," JAMA Nov. 3, 1923, 81(18):1541-1544 (an expose of a diploma mill handing our chiropractic and other degrees, reported in the section "Propaganda for Reform").

32. JAMA Feb. 3, 1912, 58(5):360-362 (reprints of mail exchanges between fake potential applicants to chiropractic school and the admission staffs of these schools, published in the "Propaganda for Reform" section. The "applicants" are made out to be fairly uneducated people, able to write but with poor spelling and grammar and with dubious motives for entering the schools. The replies of the admissions staffs assure the applicants of their ability to enter the school after sending the specified fees). See also JAMA Mar. 10, 1923, 80(10):715-716.

33. JAMA April 11, 1914, 62(15):1177 (in "Current Comment" section).

34. JAMA Mar. 3, 1917, 68(9):732 (in "Social Medicine, Medical Economics and Miscellany" section).

35. JAMA Nov. 6, 1920, 75(19):1276 (in "Current Comment").

36. JAMA Nov. 3, 1923, 81(18):1493 (a "filler" item, over 200 words).

37. JAMA Nov. 1, 1924, 83(18):1435 (in "Current Comment").

38. BMSJ July 22, 1915, 173(4):145-147.

39. BMSJ Dec. 15, 1921, 185(24):725.

40. BMSJ Dec. 29, 1921, 185(26):725.

41. BMSJ Apr. 3, 1924, 190(14):610.

42. BMSJ Nov. 8, 1923, 189(19):717.

43. For example, see BMSJ Apr. 17, 1924, 190(16):676.

44. BMSJ Oct. 2, 1924, 191(14):653.

45. BMSJ Dec. 15, 1921, 185(24):725-726.

46. JAMA May 23, 1908, 50(21)1715 (in "Medical Economics").

47. For examples, see the following issues of JAMA:
Feb. 23, 1912, 58(5):360 (in "Propaganda for Reform");
July 26, 1913, 61(4):284 (in "Current Comment," refers to chiropractic's "appeal to the cupidity of the ignorant");
Aug. 17, 1918, 71(7):571, in "Current Comment," refers to "a credulous public" and says "It is high time that the sick should be protected from such dangerous incompetents and that those who prey on the afflicted ... should be prosecuted for taking money under false pretenses.");
Oct. 30, 1929, 75(18):1209 (in "Current Comment," says "the public is not in a position to realize its grotesque nonsense.").

48. JAMA May 23, 1908, 50(21):1715.

49. See JAMA issues: Feb. 3, 1912, 58(5):360 (in "Propaganda for Reform"); Aug. 17, 1918, 71(7):571 (in "Current Comment"); and July 3, 1920, 75(1):39 (in "Current Comment").

50. Dr. Charles B. Pinkham, "The Chiropractic Problem," JAMA Apr. 2, 1921, 76(14):938 ("Association News" section).

51. BMSJ Jan. 10, 1924, 190(2):77-78; NEJM Aug. 11, 1932, 207(6):284-286.

52. For example, see BMSJ Oct. 25, 1923, 189(17):625-626; BMSJ Mar. 13, 1924, 190(11)476-477.

53. For example, see the following items in JAMA:
June 20, 1908, 50(25):2077 (in "Medical Economics;" defeat of a chiropractic bill in Oklahoma);
July 29, 1911, 57(5):412-413 (in "Medicolegal;" Missouri Supreme Court rules that chiropractic does fall under the state's medical practice act so a chiropractor's conviction is affirmed);
Mar. 7, 1914, 62(10):801 (in "Medicolegal;" Wisconsin Supreme Court rules that chiropractic does fall under the state's medical practice act so a chiropractor's conviction is affirmed);
June 9, 1917, 68(23):1704 (in "Current Comment;" discusses means by which chiropractors' attempt to have legislation passed in their favor);
Jan. 22, 1921, 76(4):254-255 in ("Medical News;" bill before Senate proposes Board of Chiropractic Examiners for Washington, D.C.);
Apr. 26, 1924, 82(17):1366 (in "Current Comment;" false story circulated that New York Medical Society had agreed to compromise legislation to license chiropractors).

54. For example, see BMSJ articles on New York (Apr. 20, 1922, 186(16):356; Apr. 3, 1924, 190(14):610) and California (Feb. 16, 1922, 186(17):229).

55. BMSJ May 19, 1921, 184(20):526-527.

56. Other examples of references to chiropractic as a trade and not a profession can be found in the "Current Comment" quotes below:

"Chiropractic is in no sense a profession." (JAMA Apr. 11, 1914, 62(15):1178).
"[W]e use the word 'trade' advisedly..." (JAMA Aug. 23, 1919. 73(8):615).
"*The Journal* has always held that 'chiropractic' is a trade and not a profession..." (JAMA Nov. 6, 1920, 75(19):1276).

57. JAMA Aug. 26, 1916, 67(9):686 (in "Current Comment").
58. JAMA Jan. 15, 1921, 76(3):184 (in "Current Comment").
59. JAMA Jan. 15, 1921, 76(3):184 (in "Current Comment").
60. JAMA Feb. 5, 1921, 76(6):385 (in "Current Comment").
61. JAMA Apr. 29, 1922, 78(17):1318 (in "Current Comment").
62. JAMA May 17, 1924, 82(20):1613 (in "Current Comment").
63. JAMA Mar. 3, 1917, 68(9):732.
64. BMSJ Dec. 15, 1921, 185(24):725.
65. BMSJ May, 19, 1921, 184(20):526-527.
66. BMSJ Jan. 10, 1924, 190(2):77-78.
67. NEJM May 2, 1929, 203(18):943-944.
68. JAMA Aug. 22, 1896, 27(8):439.
69. JAMA Apr. 4, 1896, 26(4):683.
70. JAMA Apr. 4, 1896, 26(4):683.
71. JAMA July 15, 1899, 33(3):153.
72. JAMA Oct. 7, 1899, 33(15) 922.
73. JAMA Nov. 3, 1900, 35(18) 1161.
74. JAMA Feb. 2, 1901, 36(5):329.
75. JAMA Feb. 3, 1912, 58(5) 360.
76. JAMA Apr. 11, 1914, 62(15):1177.
77. See JAMA May 25, 1895, 24(21) 811-813. In this 1895 editorial entitled "The Social Position of the Medical Profession" the author begins by chastening those who complain about the low position of medicine. The editorial proceeds to challenge the notion that physicians are not of high social position saying, "As to the doctor's social position, it is not evident that he ever had to sit at the lower end of the table" (p. 812). There follows a long listing (over 500 words) of famous upper-class physicians in history and in the present time both here in the States and in England. The author then asserts that the average physician also holds a high social position:

> The rank and file of the medical profession in this country hold a most powerful position. Some of the most enviable places in life that one ever sees are held by family doctors in good towns....(p. 812).

78. "Lay Distrust and Enmity of the Medical Profession," JAMA Oct. 24, 1896, 27(17):918-919.
79. JAMA Nov. 14, 1896, 27(20):1069.
80. JAMA Jan. 9, 1897, 28(2):86.
81. JAMA June 20, 1896, 26(25):1233-1234.
82. I am here relying upon Freidson's (1970) structural conception of medical dominance. He discusses medical dominance as a form of "organized autonomy," noting that such autonomy is protected by formal institutions and "is sustained by the dominance of its expertise in the division of labor" (1970, p. 136). Says Freidson

(1970, p. 137):
> [T]he dominant profession stands in an entirely different structural relationship to the division of labor than does the subordinate profession... In essence the difference reflects the existence of a hierarchy of institutionalized expertise.

In *The Profession of Medicine* (1971, p. 5) Freidson calls this the "preeminence" of the medical profession and notes that it was not achieved until the 20th century.

83. JAMA Feb. 8, 1896, 26(6):283.

84. JAMA Sept. 29, 1900, 35(13) 828-829.

85. JAMA Aug. 8, 1896, 27(6):329. The focus of this editorial is the patent medicine industry, although Homeopaths and antivivisectionists are also mentioned.

86.

Publication Year	Items Relating to Legal Regulation of Chiropractic
1912	1 out of 3
1913	4 out of 5
1914	4 out of 5
1915	3 out of 5
1916	4 out of 6
1917	4 out of 6
1918	4 out of 6
1919	3 out of 5
1920	3 out of 7
1921	9 out of 18
1922	7 out of 16
1923	1 out of 10
1924	4 out of 12

87. JAMA Aug. 20, 1921, 77(8):627-628.

88. Some of the assertions made in this editorial are questionable. For example, the editorial implies that chiropractors are losing all the court cases regarding the legality of their practice. But even a perusal of the cases that are reviewed in JAMA's own Medicolegal Abstracts during this period indicates that this was not so. An examination of chiropractic licensure laws shows no states licensed chiropractors until Arkansas in 1915 (Kansas passed its licensing law two years earlier, but it had not yet gone into effect or issued any licenses), thirty-nine states gave chiropractors some form of legal recognition by 1931 (Turner 1934). But these laws did limit the practice of chiropractic. Treatment modalities were generally very narrowly delimited (frequently "by hand only"). Other laws increased the educational requirements for chiropractors, although existing chiropractors were usually "grandfathered in" under this legislation (Wardwell 1982). Both the narrowing of the legal scope of chiropractic and the increase in educational requirements for chiropractors represented "victories" for orthodox medicine. But they were limited victories compared to a total victory in which chiropractic would be outlawed and a Pyrrhic victory in that the legislation (particularly the increase in educational requirements) may have significantly contributed to the ultimate survival of chiropractic.

89. JAMA April 24, 1915, 44(17):1431.

90. JAMA Dec. 25, 1915, 65(26):2228-2229.

91. JAMA Mar. 10, 1923, 80(10):715.

92. When the subordinate group expresses outrage at the dominant group it seems, at least in Western cultures, to be limited to situations where the dominant group has violated expectations of *noblesse oblige*.

Chapter 4

Solidifying Opposition, 1925 - 1960: Chiropractic as Irritant

> In the progress of medicine there is no need for the cults. The claims for chiropractic are unsound.... The history of the rise and fall of the cults is impressive. They come and go. Scientific medicine must be the resource of the future.
>
> Editorial in the *New England Journal of Medicine*, 1931[1]

By the mid-1920s, orthodox medicine has basically achieved unity within its own ranks, has achieved dominance in the medical arena and the status of physicians has been improved.[2] From 1925 to 1960, organized medicine is engaged in a process of solidifying that dominance; that is, it is involved in maintaining dominance and expanding some areas of dominance. In this context, chiropractic is seen more as an irritant than a challenge. The need for a clear rallying point to increase medicine's unity, status and dominance is no longer there. Thus, although chiropractic still exists and is solidifying *itself* as an occupational group during this time period, orthodox medicine no longer opposes chiropractic with the intensity it did during the early part of this century. Indeed, as the quotation above indicates, the demise of chiropractic is assumed.

This second phase of organized medicine's reaction to chiropractic, from 1925 to 1960, is characterized by persistent but low-level opposition to chiropractic. The opposition is most often expressed in informational updates about chiropractic, which tend to be negative reports such as convictions of chiropractors, failures of attempts to expand chiropractic practice laws, and so forth. The editorials or special expose-type reports about chiropractic that occurred so often earlier in the century are rarely seen in this period. In this section I argue that this change in the intensity and vigor of opposition to chiropractic is due to the changes in the organization and status of orthodox medicine rather than any change in chiropractic.

The efforts of orthodox medicine to solidify its dominance can be divided into two areas. First, there is occupational dominance, the efforts of orthodox medicine to solidify its dominance in the field of medicine. Secondly, there is organizational dominance, the efforts of the AMA to solidify its dominance over physicians. In both areas, however, it appears that chiropractic plays a much less important role in the maintenance or solidification of this dominance than it did in the previous period of emerging dominance. I think the reason for this is clear. During the first period, organized orthodox medicine was quite successful in forging what Burrows called its "alliance with the law." That is, organized medicine forged a link to state institutions controlling the licensing of medical practice that was essential to medical dominance. Forging this link was the difficult task and organized medicine's efforts to denigrate chiropractic were an important part of this task. During the second period, however, with that link already in place, it remained only to solidify and maintain the now legally-supported dominance. This was a much easier task. The routine publication of reports of various chiropractic "failures" in medical journals constituted an affirmation of medical dominance. When chiropractic seriously challenged this domination (such as in the case of Massachusetts in the early 1930s, when chiropractors got enough signatures from the general public to put medical practice legislation on the ballot), medical reaction was swift and intense. But for the most part, chiropractic is treated as an irritant.

The AMA's posture toward chiropractic between 1925 and 1960 thus primarily appears to be one of solidifying the opposition to chiropractic. This period is not homogenous, however, and the years 1936 to 1942 stand out as a phase of activity in some ways more similar to the first period. This spurt of activity will be discussed later in the chapter. But overall, the AMA takes a relatively passive defensive stance vis-a-vis chiropractic during this period as opposed to the more active, offensive position evidenced in the first and third periods in this century. Chiropractic is an irritant, to be persistently swatted and slapped in the knowledge that the irritant is not long for this world

THE REACTION OF MEDICINE TO CHIROPRACTIC

The Manner of Presentation of Chiropractic-Related Material in Medical Publications

From 1925 to 1960 the references to chiropractic that appear in the pages of JAMA and other medical publications are usually in the form of updates on legislation and legal rulings. These reports are typically very brief and very routine and by their brevity and repetitiveness declare chiropractic to be an irritant, but not a major concern, for organized medicine.

Continual Reports of Legislative Updates The period begins with a tremendous increase in the material being published in JAMA in regard to chiropractic, reaching a peak in 1928 with 37 items published. This increase can be primarily accounted for by the increase in the number of very brief items reported in the "Medical News" section of this journal (see figure 1 and table 1 in appendix B). For the most part, items in this section are straightforward reports from the various states which either indicate the status of proposed state legislation or report the conviction of chiropractors for practicing medicine without a license. For example, typical items in the "Medical News" section during this period read:

State Board for Registration in Chiropractic.- According to the *New England Journal of Medicine*, the newspapers reported, October 20, that chiropractors were about to file an initiative petition seeking passage of a law for the establishment of a state board of registration in chiropractic. This board would consist of three persons to be appointed by the governor to pass on the qualifications of applicants desiring to practice as chiropractors.[3]

Chiropractor and Druggist Fined.- Mrs. R.E. Lang, Portland, chiropractor, was found guilty of practicing medicine without a license by a circuit court jury, January 12. Mrs. Lang was convicted in the district court, Nov.1, 1927, fined $150, and sentenced to ten days in the county jail; she appealed to the circuit court, and Judge Stevenson affirmed the sentence of the lower court.   Mrs. Lang administered various medicines to a patient who subsequently died....[4]

Chiropractic Legal Decisions   The abundance of "Medical News" reporting diminishes quickly and by the 1930s the predominant type of item published in JAMA is the "Medicolegal Abstracts" of court cases involving chiropractors. A majority of these cases involve the interpretation of state medical practice acts in cases where chiropractors have appealed convictions for practicing medicine without a license. Like the "Medical News" items, these reports are relatively straightforward accounts of the cases. For example, a typical item in the "Medicolegal Abstracts" section reads as follows:

> Medical Practice Acts: Chiropractic as the Practice of Medicine.- Three chiropractors were convicted of violating the medical practice act of Texas. They appealed to the court of criminal appeals, which in each case held that the complaint was sufficient and that the evidence justified the judgment of conviction.... In the Langford case, the defendant admitted that he had lived in Brownwood for six years and had been a chiropractor all that time. The evidence showed that he visited a named patient and gave him "a little adjustment and rubbed his jaw - and the back of his neck." The defendant admitted making the visit and that he received $2 as a fee. This evidence was held sufficient to sustain the conviction.[5]

The reader can obtain a sense of the types of cases being published from table 2 in appendix B, which provides a list of titles of the first medicolegal abstract relating to chiropractic in each of the years comprising this second period.

With the exception of the years between 1936 and 1942, then, this period is characterized by rather colorless but negative and continuous coverage of chiropractic. The quantity of items published peaks in 1928 and greatly declines after 1952. The overall tone of this period appears to be one of dogged determination; there is persistent passive opposition to and monitoring of chiropractic activities (especially legislation) without much evidence of active opposition or commentary aimed at motivating active opposition.

The Substance of Chiropractic-Related Material in Medical Publications

Despite the fact that the AMA appears to take a relatively passive and defensive stance vis-a-vis chiropractic during this period, it is important not to lose sight of the fact that this period does appear to be one of solidifying opposition to chiropractic. While the colorful, vituperative language of the early period is absent, chiropractors and chiropractic are continually portrayed in a negative light. The denunciation of chiropractic is more indirect: reports of convictions of chiropractors for various offenses; some discrediting of individual chiropractors; and reports of injuries sustained by chiropractic patients.

Reports of Convictions As noted earlier, the "Medical News" and "Medicolegal" sections in JAMA contain numerous items concerning the convictions of chiropractors for practicing medicine without a license. In those items that report the appeal of a conviction by a chiropractor, the conviction is almost always affirmed. This constant reporting of convictions of chiropractors reinforces a negative view of chiropractic and acts to solidify the sentiments of JAMA readers regarding chiropractors and the AMA's position regarding chiropractic.

Discrediting Individual Chiropractors The indirect means of placing chiropractic in a negative light in the pages of JAMA also involves the discrediting of individual chiropractors. Sometimes this is quite subtle. It may involve noting the previous low-status occupation of a chiropractor in the course of reporting some other matter, reminiscent of the earlier focus on status differentials between chiropractic and medical practitioners.[6] It may involve the reporting of non-chiropractic illegal or questionable activities by particular chiropractors. For example, a 1928 news item reports that the president of a chiropractic college was held overnight in jail for "possession of liquor."[7] A 1948 news item notes that a California medical imposter turned his "health emporium" over to chiropractors after his conviction for practicing medicine without a license.[8] Another way of discrediting chiropractors involves the reporting of chiropractors who are convicted for illegal abortions.[9]

Reports of Injuries and Deaths Attributed to Chiropractic During this second period reports of injuries or deaths attributed to chiropractic treatment appear fairly regularly in the pages of JAMA, further contributing to the negative portrayal of chiropractic. In 1925 the first full-length article appears which provides clinical evidence of injuries apparently sustained as a result of chiropractic treatment.[10] Only two other full-length articles detailing chiropractic injuries are published during this period, but reports of injuries and deaths due directly to chiropractic treatment or due to delay of orthodox treatment while under the care of a chiropractic practitioner appear in other sections of the journal (primarily under "Medical News" and "Medicolegal Reports").[11] These reports tend to be fairly colorless, reporting convictions for manslaughter or suits for negligence and malpractice without the additional commentary regarding the menace of chiropractic that appear earlier in the century. Nevertheless, they affirm a view of chiropractic treatment as ineffective and dangerous.

Limited Spheres of Active Opposition

There are, of course, exceptions to this general pattern of lack of active opposition. Reports of actions taken and reports encouraging others to take actions against chiropractic appear in three areas: state initiatives and referendums; federal legislation; and basic science legislation. Yet even in regard to these three areas, the actions against chiropractic that are reported or are encouraged in JAMA are generally of a more defensive than offensive nature.

State Initiatives and Referendums During this period chiropractors increasingly utilize state initiative and referendum processes in attempts to enact medical practice legislation favorable to chiropractic. The progress of these efforts is monitored and reported in JAMA,[12] along with occasional commentaries praising state and local medical societies or the citizenry for their effective opposition to these measures or encouraging such opposition.[13] But the stance is a defensive one: maintain the status quo in the face of chiropractic initiatives.

Federal Legislation Likewise, in terms of federal legislation regarding chiropractic, the actions reported and encouraged in the pages of JAMA tend to be reactive or defensive in nature. Efforts by chiropractors to have favorable federal legislation enacted are monitored and reported in JAMA. Any actions by the AMA in response to these chiropractic efforts are also reported. But AMA actions that are reported or are encouraged are defensive in nature; that is, they are in response to specific actions taken by chiropractors. For example, during this second period, JAMA staff report efforts by chiropractors to have their services covered under the United States Employees' Compensation Act,[14] to have veterans' chiropractic education covered under the GI Bill,[15] to have chiropractors appointed to the Veterans Administration,[16] to have chiropractic services included in any national health insurance,[17] and to permit military deferment of chiropractic students.[18] Sometimes suggestions are made as to action that AMA members can take to oppose these efforts by chiropractors to secure favorable legislation. For example, in regard to the inclusion of chiropractic services under the United States Employees' Compensation Act, JAMA commentary notes:

> Prompt and vigorous protests filed with the House Committee on the Judiciary against enactment of Representative Tolan's chiropractic bill may prevent a further dilution of the quality of medical care to which injured federal employees are entitled under the act that the bill proposes to amend.[19]

But again, these are directives for defensive rather than offensive action.

Basic Science Legislation The last major area in which some actions are reported or encouraged in JAMA during this second period is that of basic science legislation. Basic science legislation refers to state medical practice legislation which requires aspiring practitioners of the healing arts to pass examinations in basic science areas such as chemistry, anatomy, bacteriology, and physiology before being allowed to apply for licensing or practice their healing arts in the state. Basic science boards were first established in two states in 1925. By 1943 seventeen states and the District of Columbia had basic science laws. In 1948 the secretary of the Federation of State Medical Boards stated:

> the evident original purpose of enacting basic science laws as a prerequisite for licensure in the healing arts was to exclude chiropractors and other inadequately trained practitioners from being admitted to licensure.[20]

This is a commonly acknowledged interpretation of the origin of basic science legislation. An earlier JAMA editorial explains the rise of basic science boards similarly.[21] Basic Science legislation is referred to as "corrective" and the push for such legislation is perhaps not clearly categorized as either offensive or defensive type action -- even in the limited realm of states with multiple licensing boards. But it does represent an exception to the overall lack of activity reflected in the pages of JAMA during this period.

To summarize so far: the second period is best characterized as a period during which opposition to chiropractic is solidified in a fairly passive and defensive yet persistent manner. There are few reports or commentaries encouraging action by physicians against chiropractors and those that are reported are usually made in response to actions taken by chiropractors first.

Chiropractic is portrayed in a negative light by more indirect means than those used in the first period.

SOLIDIFYING DOMINANCE AND IRRITATION WITH CHIROPRACTIC

Occupational Dominance in the Medical Arena

Organized medicine worked to further extend and solidify its newly acquired dominance in the medical arena throughout this second period. Most effort was directed to the continuing attempt to restrict the practice of medicine by raising educational standards and modifying licensing procedures. Some effort at solidifying dominance was also directed at the American public, convincing the public that orthodox medicine was the only legitimate source of health care and information. In both of these efforts, chiropractic plays an identifiable but small role.

The push for basic science legislation during the late 1920s and 1930s was an extension of the earlier single-board strategy to increase standards for health practitioners through testing. A 1929 JAMA editorial on the recently released statistics on the State Board Examinations offers the following account of this push:

> [L]egislatures have been induced to grant separate boards of examiners to osteopaths, chiropractors and certain other groups of practitioners. In each of six states which have severed such boards, *an attempt at correction* has been made through creation of basic science boards before which all applicants for licensure are required to pass before they can be admitted to the professional examination of any board.... Of course, such boards are unnecessary in states having single boards which pass on all candidates seeking authority to practice the healing art. In states having multiple boards, however, the establishing of basic science boards appears to be advisable.[22] (emphasis added)

In 1930, the AMA reiterated the function served by basic science boards in "checking the illegal practice of the cultists."[23] These boards served to further solidify the dominance of orthodox medicine. By 1943, seventeen states and the District of Columbia had basic science laws.

Likewise, changes enacted in the AMA's Principles of Medical Ethics in 1950 made it unethical for orthodox physicians to consult with non-orthodox practitioners. This acted to further restrict these practitioners and affirm the superiority of orthodox physicians. The new code read:

All voluntarily associated activities with cultists are unethical. Consultation with a cultist is a futile gesture if the cultist is assumed to have the same high grade of knowledge as is possessed by the doctor of medicine.[24]

The previous code, which had been in effect for about forty years, had simply said that "a physician should not base his practice on an exclusive dogma or sectarian system."

Efforts to restrict the legal definitions of non-orthodox practitioners continued during this second period, from 1925 to 1960. In regard to chiropractic, this primarily occurred through the efforts of local and state medical groups that organized to oppose state chiropractic initiatives and referendums instigated by chiropractors.

The period from 1925 to 1960 was also one in which the orthodox medical profession worked to solidify its image with the public as the only legitimate source of health information and care. In 1923 the AMA started publishing *Hygeia* (called *Today's Health* since 1950), a health magazine for lay audiences. In the mid-1930s the AMA began regular radio broadcasts on two national broadcasting systems (Columbia Broadcasting System and the National Broadcasting Company). The purpose of these programs was to educate the public. Medical physicians spoke on topics such as "Keeping Your Health," "The Health of the School Child," and "Progress of Medicine."[25] It is clear, however, that these broadcasts also served to reinforce the notion among the listeners that orthodox physicians are the experts in matters of health. The AMA also established a Speakers Bureau to provide presentations on medical topics to all types of groups and associations. The Bureau of Health Education provided curricular materials on health to schools. Freidson (1970) has suggested that such health education programs in schools are an institutionalized form of public relations for orthodox medicine.

Solidifying Organizational Dominance: The AMA

The AMA was busy solidifying its own position during the years from 1925 to 1960. Having achieved its goal of unity in the Progressive Era, it continues to expand its influence during the next three decades. Writing in 1941, Garceau notes that the AMA (through its link to state medical societies) exercised important controls over U.S. physicians. For example, expulsion from the societies meant no referrals and no malpractice insurance. In 1954, Hyde and colleagues note other problems for physicians that lacked membership in the AMA: they were not eligible for specialty board exams, were denied access to most hospitals, and were likely to be denied any reciprocal licensing applications. By the mid 1950s, "[I]t is only the established physician with guaranteed tenure on hospital staffs and specialty boards, or one who has the security of a faculty or governmental position who can afford to challenge the AMA" (Hyde and Wolff 1954, p. 953).

Furthermore, the power of the AMA and its affiliated state and local medical societies was enhanced by legislation that gave these societies the right to appoint the members of state boards of health and other health regulatory agencies and used AMA-determined standards for medical education and practice. By the 1950s, "the political authority of the state itself has in effect been delegated to organized medicine" (Hyde and Wolff 1954, p. 959). Organized medicine controlled the supply of physicians through its control of medical education and the conditions of medical practice and fee payment through its code of ethics.

Membership figures reflect the growing strength of the AMA during this second period. Whereas 50% of physicians were members of the AMA in 1912, by 1922 this had increased to 60% and by 1940 it had increased to 67% (Garceau 1941, p. 130).

A Brief Echo of Earlier Outrage: 1936 to 1942

There is one other feature of this second phase of medicine's opposition to chiropractic that must be discussed: the matter of the years 1936 to 1942. In some respects these years represent an exception to the overall pattern of persistent but low-level opposition to chiropractic that otherwise characterizes this second period. There were several items published during the years 1936 to 1942 that include once again the colorful language and efforts to make chiropractic look dangerous and ridiculous. It strikes one as an echo of the vituperative opposition to chiropractic earlier in the century. Indeed, I argue that this opposition reflects the issues of unity, status and domination that once again have become problematic for medicine as interest in prepaid group practice and national health insurance grows.

A few illustrations from these years are in order. In 1936 the AMA Judicial Council, in explaining the ethical proscription against professionally associating with chiropractors and other "irregulars," refers to such consultations as "degrading."[26] The response to a "Letter to the Editor" refers to chiropractic as the "illegitimate offspring of an illegitimate offspring of medicine."[27] One editorial refers to chiropractic as being "foisted" on the public and to the "inanity" of chiropractic theory.[28] Another refers to the "utter absurdity" and "ridiculous" fallacies" of chiropractic theory.[29] What can account for this brief echo of the medical outrage observed earlier in the century?

In 1932 the famous Committee on the Cost of Medical Care (CCMC) issued its final report. This committee, whose membership Odin Anderson (1982, p. 94) says "read like a who's who in health services public policy" and included fourteen physicians in private practice as well as other health personnel, issued a majority report that recommended the abandonment of solo fee-for-service medicine in favor of prepaid group practice. The minority report recommended that the private practice of medicine remain at the core of the health services system -- with the general practitioner as the cornerstone -- and that any insurance plan must be controlled by the physicians (via the medical societies). The AMA, of course, endorsed the minority report of the CCMC.[30]

The CCMC proposed no particular implementation scheme for its recommendations (Anderson 1985) and so there was no immediate concrete threat to the profession of medicine. The CCMC report, in documenting the problems faced by many Americans without the means to secure health care, did provide the basis for proponents of a national comprehensive health program in the ensuing years. These proposals *were* perceived as a concrete threat. The first National Health Survey (conducted in late 1935 to early 1936) also documented problems of financial access to health care.

President Roosevelt had appointed a Committee on Economic Security in 1934 to advise on the formulation of a Social Security program. This committee recommended that health insurance not be included in the program and the Social Security Act that passed in 1935 included no such provisions. In 1937, however, the President convened a Technical Committee on Medical Care. That committee recommended in 1938 that the government become more involved in providing health care programs, including hospital construction, child and maternal health programs, medical service for the medically indigent and a state-operated "general program of medical care" (quoted in Anderson 1985, p. 114; see also Starr 1982, p. 276). The President convened the first National Health Conference in 1938 to discuss the recommendations of this Technical Committee and those who attended generally supported that committee's recommendations. In 1939 Senator Robert Wagner introduced a health insurance bill in the Senate that was based on the recommendations of the National Health Conference. Similar bills were submitted in subsequent years: the Caper Bill in 1941; the Eliot Bill in 1942; and the Wagner-Murray-Dingell Bill in 1943 and again in 1945 (Anderson 1985, pp. 114-5).

There is also evidence of dissent among physicians over the issue of tax-supported medical insurance plans. For example, the Committee of Physicians for the Improvement of Medicine, formed in 1936, argued that health was a "direct concern of the government" (quoted in Starr 1982, p. 274), urging that the government must become involved in medical education, research, public health, and health services for the poor. The committee also favored the group practice of medicine. In 1941 the Physician's Forum was created in New York to promote national compulsory health insurance (Litman and Robins 1984, p. 348).

During these years the AMA and constituent medical societies were also involved in legal action over the AMA's attempts to fight prepaid group practice. In 1939 a U.S. Court of Appeals ruled in favor of Group Health Association, Inc. in Washington, D.C. The AMA and the District of Columbia Medical Society were then charged with attempting to restrict trade in violation of the Sherman Antitrust Act.[31]

In summary, the profession of medicine was facing a number of issues that rendered -- or potentially could have rendered -- the unity, status and dominance of medicine more problematic.

The brief burst of more intense opposition to chiropractic during this otherwise "quiet" period from 1925 to 1960 is not the result of any intentional decision to use chiropractic as a scapegoat or as a diversionary tactic of some sort. Rather, the increased efforts to stigmatize chiropractic are an integral part of the process of maintaining the occupational control and dominance that had been so recently secured by the medical profession. Just as analysis of the medical literature earlier in the century revealed a link between chiropractic and the quest for increased medical unity, status, and dominance, so too do we see this link in the medical publications from 1936 to 1942.

The proceedings of the Thirty-Third Annual Congress on Medical Education and Licensure, published in JAMA in 1937, include a broad spectrum of concerns that link again the issues of unity, status dominance and the opposition to chiropractic and other "cultist" practitioners. For example, Dr. Edward Cary speaks to all of these issues in a speech entitled "Medical Licensure as It Relates to the Practice of Medicine." I have reprinted a rather long portion of this speech because it illustrates so many concerns:

> Practitioners in recent years have become acutely conscious of impending legislation affecting their interest. Medicine today in this country would be in a sad plight if it were not organized. Eternal vigilance is required with respect to the many laws and bills touching on medicine and the methods of medical practice. It is impossible to know what political implications may be

projected by laymen who are concerned about the methods of practice of medicine. There are those who have manifested a tendency to determine for the profession and the people just what innovations are best. The medical profession has resisted this idea. It believes that in an orderly manner the leaders of medicine, who in a democratic way have had placed on their shoulders such responsibility, will be able to determine the consensus of the profession. Those appointed men reflect the general attitude of the profession of medicine toward proposed variations in medical practice. We believe, too, that a solution for the multiple economic and social problems confronting medicine can be ascertained only after consistent and open-minded study of the problems on the part of those leaders deeply interested in conditions as they exist and as they know they should exist in this mechanical or technological age. It is untrue that the medical profession is resisting an orderly transition in its relationship to society. But only through the advantages of their vast experience and knowledge of human needs and a careful analysis of the social problems can medical leaders point out advisable changes in the interest of both profession and the people.[32]

Dr. Cary then goes on to talk about the issue of physician drug addicts and how the medical profession as a whole and the boards of licensure must cooperate to eliminate these practitioners. It is interesting that he begins and ends this sensitive discussion with references to cultists. "[P]oorly equipped practitioners, particularly the cultists, succeeded only in the cities," he begins; he ends by saying "The boards of medical licensure are primarily concerned in protecting the people against illegal practitioners and quacks."[33] The passages quoted above include references to medical organization and consensus, the assertion of medical superiority over laymen, as well as references to the many problems facing medicine and the cultists. Here again we see the link between the problems faced by medicine (internally and externally) and medicine's opposition to chiropractic. This is also seen when one looks at the two papers presented at this Congress following Dr. Cary's speech. The first is "The Fallacy of Spinal Adjustment" and reports on the impossibility of the vertebral subluxation alleged by chiropractors.[34] The second, entitled "The Doctor and the Narcotic Violator," is about physicians who are themselves narcotics violators and paints these violators as outsiders: "Thirty per cent were of foreign birth..."; "Fifty per cent of the medical schools from which graduation was reported are extinct"; and so on.[35] The juxtaposition of these two papers is notable. It is as if the discussion of a problem within medicine can only be discussed after a *real* (i.e., more serious and nonmedical) problem, such as the fallacy of chiropractic, has first been noted.

Another example comes from the JAMA section "Meeting Legislative

Problems" (from the 1939 Annual Conference of Secretaries of Constituent State Medical Associations). Here Dr. George Kress of California speaks of that state's recent well-organized and successful campaign against a chiropractic initiative. Dr. A.T. McCormack responds to this by noting medicine's control of the state legislature in his home state of Kentucky and then refers to the Association's new plan of action regarding the promotion of the private practice of medicine (which was no doubt a response to the National Health Conference in 1938 and Senator Wagner's bill in 1939). Says Kress:

> Yesterday morning I felt encouraged when I saw this splendid, practical program that is workable, that means what we mean, that says we want to preserve for the people of this country the most valuable possession they have. Besides liberty itself the most valuable possession they have is the private practice of medicine.[36]

What is significant here is how in four short sentences, the speaker moves from a response to a campaign against chiropractic to the necessity to protect the private practice of medicine.

In sum, a number of events during these years 1936 to 1942 brought the issue of occupational control -- and the constituent issues of unity, status and dominance -- to the forefront once again. The specters of prepaid group practice, government involvement in health care (particularly the possibility of a compulsory national health insurance program), and dissent within the profession of medicine over these issues challenged the unity, status, and domination so recently secured by the profession and so necessary for its continued occupational control. The intensified opposition against chiropractic is part of the effort to reassert unity, status and dominance.

The next question, of course, is why the intensified opposition to chiropractic fades after 1942, not to appear again until almost twenty years later. Here there are two developments which I suggest constitute a likely explanation. The first regards the demise of prepaid group practice as a medical challenge and the second deals with the post-World War II shift in the anti-national compulsory health insurance rhetoric of organized medicine.

As I noted above, the AMA and the District of Columbia Medical Society were convicted of antitrust violations in 1940 as a result of their efforts to restrict prepaid group practice. However, after 1939 organized medicine was able to get state-level legislative restrictions on prepaid group practice enacted in twenty-six states (Starr 1982, p. 305-6; Litman and Robins 1984, p. 347). For example, sixteen states required that any prepaid medical plan be approved by the state medical society and seventeen states required that prepaid medical plans give consumers a free choice of physician (Starr 1982, p. 306). Such requirements effectively limited (or eliminated) most prepaid group practice arrangements.

The push for national compulsory health insurance (and other plans to increase government involvement in health care) does not fade after 1942 and so cannot account for any decrease in the intensity of opposition to chiropractic after that point. What does happen after 1942, however, is a shift in organized medicine's rhetoric regarding national compulsory health insurance. Medicine enters a period of "symbolic politics" from 1943 to 1950, according to Starr (1982, p. 280). "For now compulsory health insurance became entangled in the cold war," says Starr (1982 p. 280), "and its opponents were able to make 'socialized medicine' a symbolic issue in the growing crusade against communist influence in America." President Truman supported a national compulsory health plan; he proposed a comprehensive plan in 1945 and made national health insurance a priority issue in his reelection campaign in 1948 (Starr 1982, p. 284). But the AMA successfully opposed all such efforts, in part by increasingly holding out the specter of socialized medicine. When the AMA hired the public relations firm of Whitaker and Baxter to direct its campaign against a national health plan, the firm emphasized the theme that socialized medicine was the first step toward a socialist society, adopting the slogan "The Voluntary Way Is the American Way" (Hyde and Wolff 1954, p. 1014).

The brief spurt of intensity in organized medicine's opposition to chiropractic that began in 1936 thus fades after 1942. The intensity of direct opposition toward national health insurance -- now targeting "socialism" -- increased after 1942. While it might be too simplistic to argue that the specter of socialism simply replaced the specter of chiropractic, it is a correlation that cannot be ignored. I argue that the brief increase in the opposition to chiropractic served a purpose: chiropractic (and opposition to chiropractic) provided a focal point for unity, a foil against which medicine could compare itself favorably, and a mechanism through which medicine could reassert and justify its dominance. When organized medicine successfully dealt with the problems (or potential problems) of dissension among the ranks of physicians, prepaid group practice, and, to a lesser extent, the issue of national health insurance, it once again turned away from concern with chiropractic. Organized medicine was successful in preventing the creation of any compulsory comprehensive national health program, but that struggle turned out to be more ongoing.

Conclusion: Solidifying Dominance and Chiropractic as Irritant

I think it is fair to conclude that chiropractic plays only a small role in the efforts of orthodox medicine to solidify its dominance in the medical arena during the years under consideration here, 1925 to 1960. The large numbers of items about chiropractic published in JAMA during the late 1920s, for example, are comprised mostly of one-paragraph "Medical News" items or "Medicolegal" reports that give an overall negative picture of chiropractic and its prospects. The sheer quantity and matter-of-fact tone of this reporting affirms the view of orthodox medicine as dominant. Even in the few areas where I have identified a concern with chiropractic, such as the basic science legislation and the ethical proscription against consulting with cultists, the reports are still quite neutral in tone; with the exception of the years 1936 to 1942 (discussed above), there are no vituperative diatribes such as were common in the earlier decades of this century or those seen in the later decades of the third period.

I argue that this retreat of orthodox medicine from its frenzied opposition to chiropractic makes sense in terms of the framework of interpretation that I have outlined at the beginning of this book and this chapter. The orientation of orthodox medicine to chiropractic is not merely a response to alleged scientific inadequacies of chiropractic or even a response to the perceived increase or decrease in the efficacy of chiropractic as a medical competitor. Orthodox medicine's orientation to chiropractic is an integral part of its own development as an occupation and thus reflects the functional needs of this occupation as it responds to changing external circumstances (affecting occupational dominance in the medical arena) and internal circumstances (the organizational dominance of the AMA). Orthodox medicine's orientation to chiropractic is part of the reality that is socially constructed by orthodox medicine in its publications to its own members and the general public.

An examination of some alternative hypotheses is in order. I discard the *scientific hypothesis* explaining orthodox medicine's rejection of chiropractic -- that orthodox medicine's response to chiropractic can be explained by the scientific inadequacies of chiropractic theory and practitioners. As I have already noted, such an hypothesis predicts a consistent level of rejection of chiropractic which the evidence does not bear out.

A second hypothesis, the *medical competitor hypothesis*, links orthodox medicine's orientation to chiropractic to the real competitive threat posed by chiropractic. With this hypothesis, the observation of the decreased intensity of orthodox medicine's opposition to chiropractic during the 1925 to 1960 period under discussion would lead to a prediction that this decrease was a result of the decreased threat posed by chiropractic. Again the evidence does not bear this out. The data on numbers of chiropractors during this period indicates a fairly stable or slowly growing body of chiropractic practitioners during this period. Wardwell reports that there were an estimated 16,000 practicing chiropractors in 1929[37] and 23,000 qualified to practice in 1960 (Wardwell 1982, p. 219; 1963, p. 216).

Chiropractic also made progress in the quality of its educational programs during this period. John J. Nugent, Director of Education of the NCA, traveled the country advocating that "smaller schools must merge, all schools must teach '4 years of 4,' all institutions must become non-profit, professionally-owned, and curriculums must be standardized, faculties strengthened and clinical opportunities expanded" (Gibbons, as quoted in Wardwell 1982, p. 218). In 1930, shortly before Nugent began his crusade, there were 42 chiropractic schools, almost all proprietary, teaching a course at least 18 months long. National College of Chiropractic was the first to implement the 4-year chiropractic curriculum and by the 1950s, the 4-year course had become the rule (Gibbons 1977, p. 146).

By 1931, thirty-nine states gave legal recognition to chiropractic and even in those states that did not, chiropractors continued to practice. Massachusetts, for example, was a state considered unfriendly to chiropractors and did not license chiropractors until 1974. However, Wardwell (1982 p. 226) notes that in 1950 there were nonetheless 250 to 300 practicing chiropractors in that state.

In-patient chiropractic hospitals also emerged during this period. In 1928 Hariman Hospital was built in North Dakota and the Spears Chiropractic Hospital opened in Denver during World War II. Gibbons reports the "[c]hiropractic hospitals and sanitariums existed, if not flourished, for most of the period from 1920 to 1960" and there were close to a hundred in-patient chiropractic hospitals existing up until World War II (Gibbons 1980, p. 16). But this second period also saw the decline of these facilities, perhaps, as Gibbons suggests, because they were all built and operated without federal money and at that time few patients were covered by private insurance policies and few private policies covered chiropractic care.

Chiropractic did suffer some setbacks during the early part of this period.[38] But it is difficult to argue that chiropractic posed a significantly decreased threat to organized medicine in the years 1925 to 1960 than it did in the years preceding this period (assuming it was ever a threat at all).

A third alternative hypothesis, the *perceived medical competitor hypothesis*, proposes that the response of orthodox medicine to chiropractic can be accounted for by the perception of chiropractic as a threat to orthodox medicine. This hypothesis suggests that -- regardless of the objective threat or lack thereof posed by chiropractic -- a decrease in the perception of chiropractic as a threat can explain the decreased intensity of response during this second period. Certainly there is some evidence that the ascendance of orthodox medicine is assumed to be inevitable and that chiropractic, like the other cults and sects, will surely decline. "After all, " reads an editorial in NEJM, "we find nothing but the old, old story, the exploiting of the suggestibility of humanity, under a new name and by a device that in time will pass into limbo with the metallic tractors of Dr. Elisha Perkins."[39]

There are those who argue further that chiropractic is indeed on the decline, such as the Massachusetts physician who notes that it would be foolish to set up a separate examining board for a medical sect, especially "if the sect is shrinking so rapidly as is chiropractic, on which as a sect the hand of death is already visible."[40]

This third hypothesis is more difficult to test since the diminished intensity of response to chiropractic during this period means there is much less written about chiropractic at all during this second period. I think it is clear, however, that chiropractic is not perceived as a threat to orthodox medicine during this second period. Indeed, as I have argued in this chapter, throughout most of this period chiropractic is seen as an irritant, not a threat. But if chiropractic is considered less of a threat during this period *it is only because of the increasingly dominant position of medicine*, not a corresponding diminishment in the position of chiropractic.

NOTES

1. NEJM Apr. 9, 1931, 204(15):783.
2. Starr (1982, pp.142-143) reports data that indicates that physicians' incomes improved dramatically between 1900 and 1928. Even by the most conservative measure, he says that their incomes quadrupled (whereas prices only doubled). He also notes that the prestige of physicians rose significantly.
3. JAMA Nov. 14, 1931, 97(20):1472 ("Medical News-Massachusetts").
4. JAMA Feb. 18, 1928, 90(7):553 ("Medical News-Oregon").
5. JAMA Apr. 22, 1939, 112(16):1633. Hoy v. State (Texas), 115 S.W. (2d) 629; Ehrke v. State (Texas), 115 S.W. (2d) 631; Langford v. State (Texas), 115 S.W. (2d) 632.

6. For example, see JAMA Aug. 18, 1928, 91(7):505 ("Medical News-New York"). This is a report of a patient dying in a chiropractor's office. In referring to the chiropractor, the report notes: "He is a carpenter by trade."

7. JAMA Feb. 25, 1928, 90(8):622 ("Medical News-California").

8. JAMA Oct. 23, 1948, 138(8):60 ("Medical News-California").

9. See "Medical News" items in the following JAMA issues: June 2, 1928, 90(22):1797 ("Minnesota"); Jan. 5, 1929, 92(1):62 ("Maine"); May 4, 1929, 92(18):1526 ("California"); July 6, 1929, 93(1):39 ("California"); Oct. 6, 1934, 103(14):1075 ("Minnesota"); Sept. 3, 1938, 111(10):948-9 ("Minnesota"); Jan. 17, 1942, 118(3):239 ("Minnesota"); Nov. 7, 1942, 120(10):775 ("Minnesota"); Feb. 20, 1943, 121(8):609 ("Minnesota"); Nov. 11, 1944, 126(11):714 ("California"); and Mar. 24, 1945, 127(12):724 ("Minnesota").

10. Edward S. Blaine, "Manipulative (Chiropractic) Dislocations of the Atlas," JAMA Oct. 31, 1925, 85(18):1356-1359.

11. H.R. Pratt-Thomas and Knute E. Berger, "Cerebellar and Spinal Injuries after Chiropractic Manipulation," JAMA Mar. 1, 1947, 133(9):600-603; David Green and Robert J. Joynt, "Vascular Accidents to the Brainstem Associated with Neck Manipulation," JAMA May 30, 1959, 170(5):522-524. Individual references to other items (besides the full-length articles cited above) reporting injury resulting form chiropractic treatment are too numerous to cite. However, the numbers of such items appearing in JAMA during five-year intervals of this period are listed below. All items appear in the "Medical News" or "Medicolegal" sections of the journal, except for one item each appearing in "Current Comment," "Foreign Letters," and "Correspondence."

Years	Number of Items
1925-1929	14
1930-1934	2
1935-1939	6
1940-1944	9
1945-1949	3
1950-1954	3
1955-1959	2
1960-1961	0

12. See "Medical News" items in the following issues of JAMA: Oct. 1, 1927, 89(14):1159 ("Ohio"); Nov. 5, 1927, 89(19):1614 ("Ohio"); Nov. 12, 1927, 89(20):1701 ("Ohio"); Nov. 14, 1931, 97(20):1472 ("Massachusetts"); Oct. 22, 1932, 99(17):1437 ("Massachusetts"); Nov. 19, 1932, 99(21):1787 ("Arizona"); Nov. 19, 1932, 99(21):1788 ("Massachusetts"); Oct. 27, 1934, 103(17):1314 ("California"); Dec. 1, 1934, 103(22):1713 ("California"); Apr. 30, 1938, 110(18):1466 ("Reports of Officers"); and June 5, 1954, 155(6):585 ("Washington").

13. See JAMA "Editorial" and "Current Comment" items in the following issues: Oct. 22, 1927, 89(17):1431; Nov. 5, 1932, 99(19):1608; Nov. 19, 1932, 99(21):1785; Nov. 17, 1934, 103(20):1541; Feb. 12, 1938, 110(7):513-514; Nov. 5, 1938, 111(19):1769; and Nov. 19, 1938, 111(21):1938.

14. See JAMA issues: Mar. 30, 1940, 114(13):1270 ("Current Comment"); Apr. 19, 1941, 116(16):1798 ("Reports of Officers-Organization Section"); Apr. 25, 1942 118(17):1478 ("Reports of Officers-Organization Section"); Apr. 24, 1943, 121(17):1381 ("Reports of Officers-Organization Section"); May 27, 1944, 125(4):290 ("Organization Section"); June 9, 1945, 128(6):453 ("Medical News-New York"); and Oct. 27, 1945, 129(9):637 ("Report of Board of Trustees-Organization Section").

15. See JAMA issues: Oct. 27, 1945, 129(9):637 ("Report of Board of Trustees-Organization Section"); May 10, 1947, 134(2):167 ("Reports of Officers-Organization Section"); and May 14, 1949, 140(2):229 ("Current Comment").

16. See JAMA issues: July 31, 1926, 87(5):334-335 ("Medical News-General"); Mar. 19, 1927, 88(12):949 ("Medical Economics"); June 18, 1949, 140(7):633, ("Organization Section-Washington Letter"); July 16, 1949, 140(11):964 ("Organization Section-Washington Letter"); Feb. 10, 1951, 145(6):409 ("Organization Section-Federal Legislation"); Apr. 21, 1951, 145(16):1271 ("Organization Section-Federal Legislation"); Apr. 21, 1951, 145(16):1271 ("Organization Section-Federal Legislation"); and May 22, 1954, 155(4):369 ("Organization Section").

17. JAMA July 6, 1946, 131(10):840, 847 ("Organization Section") and JAMA July 2, 1949, 140(9):820 ("Organization Section-Washington Letter").

18. JAMA Dec. 22, 1951, 147(17):1699-1700 ("Organization Section") and JAMA June 28, 1952, 149(9):860 ("Proceedings of the Chicago Session").

19. JAMA Mar. 30, 1940, 114(13):1270 ("Current Comment").

20. JAMA May 1, 1948, 137(1):111 ("Congress on Medical Education and Licensure").

21. See Harry Eugene Kelly, "Basic Science Statutes," JAMA Aug. 17, 1929, 93(7):519, where Basic Science laws are discussed as "corrective legislation." This author says: "The fact that the claims of the cults are in truth without merit, but nevertheless are recognized by law, moves us to seek a method, indirect though it must be, of protecting the public health against the low standards of professional training advocated and established by them .... This plan has been recently developed into the existing so-called basic science statute."

Also see JAMA April 23, 1932, 98(17):1467, where the usefulness of basic science legislation for states with multiple boards is reiterated.

22. JAMA Apr. 27, 1929, 92(17):1446.

23. "Statistics and State Board Examinations," JAMA Apr. 26, 1930, 94(17):1322.

24. Code of Ethics, 1950, quoted from "How the New Ethics Code Affects You," ME Oct. 1950, 27(1):56.

25. JAMA Mar. 3, 1934, 102(9) 702.

26. JAMA Apr. 4, 1936, 106(14):1197.

27. JAMA May 6, 1939, 112(18):1853.

28. JAMA Feb.1, 1941, 116(5):414.

29. JAMA Sept. 26, 1942, 120(4):293.

30. JAMA Dec. 3, 1932, 99(23):1951.

31. JAMA May 11, 1940, 114(19):1903.

32. JAMA Apr. 10, 1937, 108(15):1284.

33. JAMA Apr. 10, 1937, 108(15):1285.

34. *Ibid.*

35. JAMA Apr. 10, 1937, 108(15):1286.

36. JAMA Jan. 13, 1940, 114(2):166.

37. Wardwell cites his source for this data as the Committee on the Costs of Medical Care (*Medical Care for the American People: Final Report of the Committee on the Costs of Medical Care*, Chicago: Chicago University Press, 1932).

38. Gibbons argues that 1924 was the peak and final year in the "Golden Age" of chiropractic and that after this "a depression in both economics and self-confidence overtook chiropractic (Gibbons 1977, p. 146). B.J. Palmer introduced the neurocalometer in that year and this instrument -- and the self-serving policies that accompanied it -- was the source of major conflict in chiropractic in the ensuing years. The professional associations split on this issue and the Palmer School itself suffered enormously. From a peak enrollment of 3100 in 1922 it declined dramatically to an enrollment of only 300 in 1929 (Gibbons 1980, p. 19). But to argue that this decline was a generalized decline for all of chiropractic is to overemphasize the role of B.J. Palmer and the Palmer School in chiropractic at that time in history. By the late 1920s numerous other chiropractic schools had arisen, frequently begun by chiropractors who disagreed with Palmer on a variety of scientific and educational issues. Many of these schools were short-lived. Some, however, became well-known centers of chiropractic education. The National College of Chiropractic, for example, was established in 1906 by John Howard, who wanted to include more human dissection in the chiropractic curriculum (Gibbons 1980). National grew to be the center of "mixer" chiropractic education in the United States and continues this distinction. It is clear that 1924 was a significant year for chiropractic, but it was not "the beginning of the end." Rather, it was the crystallizing of the major split in chiropractic (see chapter 2). And, more specifically, it marks the end of B.J. Palmer's "preeminence" in the profession (Wardwell 1982, p. 218).

39. NEJM Feb. 11, 1932, 206(6):299.

40. Stephen Rushmore, M.D., "The Bill to Register Chiropractors," NEJM Mar. 24, 1932, 206(12):614-615.

Chapter 5

The Campaign Against Chiropractic, 1961 - 1976: Chiropractic as Enemy

It is the position of the medical profession that chiropractic is an unscientific cult whose practitioners lack the necessary training and background to diagnose and treat human disease. Chiropractic constitutes a hazard to national health care in the United States because of the substandard and unscientific education of its practitioners and their rigid adherence to an irrational, unscientific approach to disease causation.

Statement of policy adopted by AMA House of Delegates in 1966

How ironic that as medicine enters the decade wherein so many changes in the organization of medical care and financing are taking place the AMA should decide to renew its attack on chiropractic. Why pour resources into the battle against chiropractic when these resources are sorely needed to address the looming Medicare debate in Congress? Why encourage members to initiate a major campaign against chiropractors when those same members are needed to lobby for traditional fee-for-service financing structures and medical control over delivery of service decisions? Yet this apparently inexplicable effort on the part of the AMA begins to make sense when one understands how the fight against chiropractic actually serves the agenda of the AMA. For in fighting chiropractic, organized medicine is serving itself and the profession: focusing on unity in the face of factionalism, demonstrating its superiority in the face of a doubting public, and reasserting its dominance in the face of bureaucratic and legislative challenges to that dominance.

So it is that during this period, from 1961 to 1976, organized medicine begins to intensify opposition to chiropractic. We see medicine taking the offensive against chiropractic in trying to have the occupation labeled "quackery" and "cultist" through a very vigorous campaign against quackery of all types and against chiropractic in particular. In fact, the stance it assumes during this period is much more similar to its position during the first decades of this century than the position taken during the preceding thirty-odd years. Again, I argue that the change in the orientation to chiropractic in this last stage is due to the changes in the position of medicine in the medical arena and in American society rather than a response to changes in chiropractic. The renewed vigor with which organized medicine pursues chiropractic is a reflection of social developments in the organization of medicine and society, *not* a reaction to developments in chiropractic. In the 1960s and 1970s medicine once again faces issues of unity, status and dominance. Of particular importance are the challenge to medicine's control over the provision of medical care and organizational setbacks in the AMA.

THE REACTION OF MEDICINE TO CHIROPRACTIC

The Manner of Presentation of Chiropractic-Related Material in Medical Publications

There are many fewer items dealing with chiropractic in the pages of JAMA during this third period, from 1961 to 1976, than appeared during the vigorous push to solidify the opposition to chiropractic in the 1920s. However, in relation to the scant attention given to chiropractic in the 1950s, we see a resurgence of items published in the 1960s and early 1970s. Furthermore, two additional relevant medical publications, the newspaper *American Medical Association News* (AMAN) and the journal *Medical Economics* (ME), begin just prior to this period in history. These two journals publish numerous items relating to chiropractic in the period under discussion. Interested readers can refer to tables 3, 4, and 5 and figure 4 in appendix B for quantitative details on the numbers and types of articles appearing in these publications.

Particularly notable is the kind of article that appears in JAMA during this period. While the predominant form of reporting appears to be the short notices (usually 100 to 300 words) appearing in the "AMAgrams" section, there are many more editorials and full-length articles than in the second period. It is this form of publication, as much as the content and numbers of items, that attests to the importance attributed to the campaign against chiropractic or at least an increase in concern about chiropractic.

The Substance of Chiropractic-Related Material in Medical Publications

There is a tremendous amount of material published about chiropractic by organized medicine after 1960. Not all the material focuses on chiropractic itself; much is written encouraging readers to influence the public and legislators to join the campaign against chiropractic and to seek organizational allies in this campaign.

The AMA Campaign against Quackery   The campaign against chiropractic was part of a larger battle against quackery of all types. In October 1961 the first National Congress on Medical Quackery was co-sponsored by the AMA and the Food and Drug Administration The director of the Legal and Socioeconomic Division of the AMA, who presided over the congress, said he hoped the conference would "be the beginning of a hard-hitting and revitalized crusade by private and governmental agencies against the hucksters of pseudomedicine."[1] A second conference was held in 1963. In 1966 the Third National Congress on Medical Quackery, this time co-sponsored by the AMA and the National Health Council, included chiropractic as a formal topic for the first time.[2] In fact, this conference began the day after a Seminar on Chiropractic Legislation was held by the AMA for the state medical societies.[3] The 1968 Fourth National Congress on Health Quackery also included sessions on chiropractic.[4]

The Focus on Chiropractic as Enemy   The push against chiropractic clearly constitutes the center of the more general campaign against quackery during this period. The AMA's Department of Investigation was begun in 1906 as the Propaganda Department, the function of which was to investigate patent medicines and other types of quackery.[5] In November 1963, the Committee on Quackery was created within the Department of Investigation and it was this committee that was responsible for much of the vigor behind the attack on chiropractic during the 1960s. According to a 1966 pamphlet put together by this committee entitled "Chiropractic: The Unscientific Cult," the Committee on Quackery was "assigned the specific mission of determining the true nature of chiropractic and its practitioners and to inform the medical profession and the public of its findings."[6]

The finding that the "true nature" of chiropractic was unscientific and a cult was no doubt a foregone conclusion given the title of the committee to which this task was assigned. However, the committee was nonetheless kept busy with these tasks. For example, in 1964, the first year of its operation, the committee published a report based on fake letters of application sent to seven chiropractic schools that concluded that chiropractic schools do not in fact require the minimum educational qualifications that they profess to require.[7] In 1965 the committee put together an exhibit called "Information on Chiropractic."[8] The committee had an especially busy year in 1966 and summarized its activities in the Annual Reports of the Committees of the Board of Trustees of the AMA as follows:

> The Third National Congress on Medical Quackery was planned for October 7-8, 1966, and the Seminar on Chiropractic Legislation for state medical societies, for October 6. A report on the "Educational Background of Chiropractic School Faculties" was included in a packet on chiropractic for distribution at the congress and seminar. Also included were a pamphlet, "Chiropractic: The Unscientific Cult," made from a slide-film documentary prepared by a committee member; an article in the September issue of the *New Physician* on "The Scientific Brief Against Chiropractic," a two-page feature article in the *AMA News* on the case of *England v. Louisiana State Board of Medical Examiners*, which upheld Louisiana's right to refuse to license chiropractic, and a survey of chiropractic licensing laws.
>
> The exhibit, "Information on Chiropractic," was shown at seven state medical society conventions and at the AMA Annual and Clinical Conventions. Assistance was given to state medical societies and numerous foreign medical associations in their opposition to proposed chiropractic legislation. The slide-film documentary on chiropractic was shown and made available to state medical society gatherings.
>
> Letters were sent to each state medical society suggesting approaches for opposing the cult of chiropractic, and to each specialty society and medical school dean on the ethical proscription against professional association with cultists. Statements were prepared urging physicians to report possible violations of state medical practice acts by chiropractors to state

medical examining boards, and alerting state medical societies to attempts by chiropractors to obtain use of hospital facilities.[9]

These are but a sampling of the activities of the committee which was the driving force behind the aggressive campaign against chiropractic during this third period.

The attack upon chiropractic appears to be three-pronged, involving efforts to influence physicians themselves, legislation, and the public. Each of these areas will be dealt with in turn, although any given activity or report may serve multiple purposes.

Influencing Physicians Efforts at influencing members of the medical profession itself appear to be the "first line" of attack in the campaign against chiropractic. Although most of what is published in JAMA simply assumes that the readership recognizes chiropractic as quackery, other items seem to be more directed at convincing the readers that this is indeed the case (or report activities which have this as their goal). I refer to these direct attempts to influence physicians as information or educational efforts. The aforementioned exhibit entitled "Information on Chiropractic" is an example of these educational efforts. This exhibit, which was a medium for distributing literature on chiropractic, traveled primarily to meetings of state medical societies, although it was also displayed at the 1965 national meetings of the AMA.[10] Notices of pamphlets and other material published by the AMA Department of Investigation are typically reported in the "AMAgrams" section of JAMA.[11]

Occasionally, direct notice is given to physicians regarding rules covering their formal interaction with chiropractors. For example, the following reminder was printed in JAMA in 1966:

> It has come to the attention of the Committee that certain groups of chiropractors in different sections of the country are seeking to apply pressure on public officials to obtain the privilege of practicing their unscientific cult in certain hospitals. The Committee reminds all state and county medical societies that chiropractors are not allowed to practice in any hospital accredited by the Joint Commission on Accreditation of Hospitals.[12]

This type of reminder was sent to medical schools and specialty societies in regards to the AMA Code of Ethics' prohibition against associating with chiropractors.[13] Notice is also given that there is no legal requirement to provide chiropractors with patient records or x-rays, as will be discussed in a later section.

In November of 1966, as a climax to the many anti-chiropractic activities that year, the AMA House of Delegates adopted for the first time a formal statement of policy on chiropractic. This statement, which is quoted in part at the beginning of this chapter, was submitted to the House by the Committee on Quackery.[14] Perhaps the adoption of this statement was more symbolic than material in intent. The position was certainly not new. However, its passage in the House indicated consensus among physicians in the condemnation of chiropractic. State and local medical societies were urged to formally endorse this statement.[15]

Influencing Legislation The AMA attempted to influence various types of legislation regarding chiropractic during this third period, particularly at the national level. Many of these actions are reported in JAMA. For example, in 1962 the AMA urged Congress not to pass legislation that would allow chiropractic services to be covered under the Federal Employees Compensation Act.[16] In 1964 the AMA testified against chiropractic before the Senate Aging Subcommittee on medical quackery.[17] In 1967 the AMA testified against inclusion of chiropractic services under Medicare Part B.[18] In 1973 the AMA testified against chiropractic associations being an accrediting agency under the Office of Education,[19] against coverage of chiropractic services under Medicare,[20] and against a proposed change in federal Motor Carrier Safety Regulations to allow chiropractors to conduct physical examinations of commercial drivers.[21]

Additionally, the AMA Committee on Quackery provided ongoing assistance to state medical societies in opposing state level legislation regarding chiropractic.[22] Physicians were urged to contact state and federal legislators regarding the dangers of chiropractic.[23]

Influencing the Public As was the case in earlier years, the offensive against chiropractic takes place within the framework of the rhetoric of safeguarding the public. Perhaps what differentiates this third period in this regard, however, is the effort to safeguard the public not only through protective legislation but by directly informing or "educating" the public about the dangers of chiropractic. This is spelled out clearly in 1966:

> The people have a right to make their own mistakes, but the medical profession has an obligation to exposed cultist practices so the people will not make this mistake unknowingly. Its obligation arises, not out of animosity toward the cultists, but from dedication to the welfare of the public.[24]

The efforts of the AMA to educate the public regarding chiropractic occurred two ways: direct contact with the public or contact via the doctor-patient connection. These activities are publicized in JAMA. The AMA made direct contact with the public through the provision of public speakers and through replies to inquiries directed to the Department of Investigation.[25]

Most of the responsibility for educating the public about chiropractic appears to have been given to physicians themselves. For example, the editorial response to a letter about chiropractors giving physical examinations for the Civil Air Patrol and Boy Scout camps was:

> [T]he local physicians have an obligation to the public to educate them to the advantages that would accrue from a complete scientific physical examination by one thoroughly trained in scientific medicine. This is an educational process which is long, slow, and arduous, but which falls on the shoulders of doctors of medicine in a situation like this.[26]

Public education through the doctor-patient connection appears to have taken place primarily through the distribution of chiropractic literature which was available from the AMA at a nominal cost (such as $10.00 for one thousand pamphlets[27]). These pamphlets were placed in doctors' waiting rooms or sent to patients with their bills.[28] Physicians were sometimes specifically asked to contact members of the public regarding chiropractic. An example of this is a 1964 editorial which directed physicians "to alert high-school students and their guidance counselors to the inadequacy of chiropractic education and to the fact that a career in chiropractic is a career in cultism."[29] Physicians whose patients were "victimized by cultist practices" were asked to encourage them to report this to the police.[30] There were also more general calls for physicians to inform the public about the problem of chiropractic.[31]

Seeking Allies in the Fight against Chiropractic In this third period, some effort is made to point out that other groups also reject chiropractic. For example, there are items that report the rejection of chiropractic by radiologists,[32] the National Council of Senior Citizens,[33] the federal Task Force on Medicaid and Related Programs,[34] the AFL-CIO,[35] the Canadian Medical Association,[36] French physicians,[37] and the American Public Health Association.[38] There is extensive coverage of the HEW report to Congress, "Independent Practitioners Under Medicare," which concluded that chiropractic services should not be covered under Medicare.[39] In fact, complimentary copies of this report were reprinted in pocket size by the AMA.[40] Likewise, the 1969 book by journalist Ralph Smith, entitled *At Your Own Risk: The Case Against Chiropractic*, was given significant attention in the pages of JAMA.[41] The AMA Department of Investigation sent 100 copies of the book to each state medical society and sent one copy to each of the 1,200 largest libraries in the country.[42] Reports of many of the above organizations are quoted in the Department of Investigation's pamphlet "What They Say About Chiropractic," which is a "compilation of antichiropractic statements made in recent years by national health and nonhealth organizations."[43] Likewise Maisel's *Reader's Digest* article was quoted extensively in an editorial[44] and Crelin's *American Scientist* article was reprinted and widely distributed by the AMA.[45]

You may recall that during the years 1908 to 1924 JAMA also occasionally reprinted others' comments regarding chiropractic. In that case the reprints seemed to be more an unwillingness to expend much effort than anything else; that is, the view was that chiropractic was too silly to expend any real energy to oppose and that it was sufficient to quote the opinions of others and "findings" of others are reprinted to bolster and affirm the AMA's position in opposing chiropractic. I have placed the word "findings" in quotations not only because this is the word used in JAMA but because the authors do not always appear to have any expert knowledge to apply to the question of chiropractic. Examples here are the reports by the AFL-CIO and the National Council of Senior Citizens which are referred to over and over again (see notes 33 and 35).

Considerable attention is given to the legal decisions affecting chiropractic during this period. The decision given the most attention is the 1965 case, affirmed by the U.S. Supreme Court in 1966, where the court ruled that Louisiana had the right to require chiropractors to have the same educational requirements as medical physicians for licensing.[46] Other legal matters reported include: that physicians are not legally obligated to furnish x-rays[47] and other medical records[48] to chiropractors who request them; that hospitals can legally deny staff privileges to chiropractors;[49] and that the New York Supreme Court upheld a law preventing chiropractors from using x-rays.[50] There are also reports of chiropractors being convicted of second degree murder[51] and manslaughter[52] of their patients and of chiropractors losing libel[53] and slander[54] suits against persons who have criticized chiropractic.

Summary In sum, this third period is characterized by a vigorous campaign against chiropractic. Towards the end of the period there appears in the pages of JAMA a sense of anger, tinged perhaps with incredulity and frustration that medicine does not appear to be winning this battle. We see editorials entitled "Put Up or Shut Up"[55] and "A Call to Arms."[56] A letter to the editor from a Missouri physician concludes:

Like many others who are tired of reading reports which now only repeat themselves, I would like to see some action.[57]

UNITY, STATUS AND DOMINANCE AND CHIROPRACTIC AS ENEMY

After more than three golden decades of enjoying a high degree of status, unity of identity and organization and dominance in the medical arena, medicine enters the 1960s facing some challenges that threaten to disrupt these hard won gains. Some of these challenges come from outside the profession and threaten the dominance and status of the profession. These are the challenges of changing medical financing, new funding mechanisms for medical education, changing institutional arrangements regarding specialization, hospitals, and HMOs, and changes in the doctor-patient relationship. Others are challenges from within the profession itself, such as the consequences of the AMA's defeat in the battle against Medicare and Medicaid, factionalism within the AMA, membership decline and financial difficulties. Each of these challenges will be discussed below. The final sections of the chapter will address how the social dynamics spawned by the opposition of organized medicine to chiropractic enabled organized medicine to better handle the internal and external challenges it faced.

Challenges to Medical Control Over Provision of Care

After more than thirty years of reigning as a "sovereign profession," as Starr (1982) phrases it, medicine faces -- and succumbs to -- several challenges beginning at the end of the 1950s, gaining momentum in the 1960s, and continuing to the present time. These challenges were posed by the federal government, by provider institutions, and by patients themselves. Changes in medical service payment, the funding of medical education, institutional arrangements, and physician-patient relationships were all part of the assault on medical status, autonomy and control over the conditions of medical work and the provision of medical care.

Payment for Medical Services Orthodox medicine (and the AMA in particular) has viewed any intervention in the doctor-patient relationship -- including the economic relationship -- as interference. The direct fee-for-service model of payment has thus been the preferred model throughout medical history in the United States and until recently the AMA has actively opposed almost all attempts to modify that model. The AMA opposed dispensaries at the turn of the century, opposed corporate medical practice during the 1920s and 1930s, and has opposed all national health service proposals since 1920. The AMA's acceptance of private "voluntary" insurance came only after it became clear that such support would be necessary to avert the possibility of any national compulsory plan and that physicians would retain control over almost all aspects of the voluntary system (Law 1974; Starr 1982).

The introduction of the Forand bill in Congress in 1957, proposing the coverage of some medical services for the elderly under the Social Security program, was ultimately expanded and passed in the Medicare and Medicaid legislation of 1965. The passage of this legislation represented a major blow to the status of medicine and to the autonomy it had enjoyed for over thirty years. It is true that the AMA and other physician groups did much to delay this legislation and to shape it into a more palatable form. But the AMA had fought this battle wholeheartedly and yet it had lost.

The AMA campaign against the King-Anderson bill in 1961 (which embodied President Kennedy's proposal for health insurance for the elderly to be covered by the Social Security program) was an "all out effort" according to David Baldwin, who worked on the campaign (quoted in Campion 1984, p. 258):

> It was an all out effort. Pamphlets? We turned them out by the thousands. We wrote public service announcements and prepared newspaper mats for the local societies. The field service staff got to work on an endorsement campaign. We had speakers' bureaus. We had prepared speeches. We had canned video talks. We had everything. *We turned on every tap that we could.* (emphasis added)

The costs of these efforts were steep, with the AMA declaring $163,404 in lobbying expenses in 1961, $83,075 in 1962, $74,457 in 1963, $45,515 in 1964 and $1,165,935 in 1965 (the last figure includes the cost of the AMA advertising campaign, according to Campion (1984, p. 25)). The AMA spent additional funds battling this legislation through its political action committee, AMPAC, which spent $709,163 between 1961 and 1964 on political campaigns for federal offices (Campion 1984, p. 259).

The 1965 Medicare and Medicaid legislation was only the beginning of federal legislation providing health care coverage for eligible elderly and poor and of regulations for the provision of such care. The Social Security Act continued to be amended in various ways, such as the 1966 amendments that relate to the quality of care in nursing homes receiving Medicare and Medicaid funds and 1972 amendments establishing Professional Standards Review Organizations (PRSOs) to oversee quality and quantity of care provided by physicians servicing patients receiving federally-funded medical care (Litman and Robins 1984). The PRSOs represented a particularly important incursion into the autonomy and control of medicine. Even though the review boards were primarily composed of physicians, and even though some argue that they had negligible effect, they still were the first external review agencies acting independently of state and local medical societies, Boards of Medical Examiners, and the AMA. Here, too, the PRSOs had been adamantly but unsuccessfully opposed by the AMA and this loss was another chink in the position of the AMA and the medical profession.

In 1966 the Office of Economic Opportunity began to formally fund comprehensive neighborhood health centers and these centers were also funded by the Department of Health, Education and Welfare under the Comprehensive Health Planning Act (Starr 1982). These programs were designed to improve health care delivery in the U.S., especially to the poor. But these programs and the numerous regulations regarding their operation represented another incursion by the federal government into the medical arena, dictating in yet another area the conditions and contexts of the provisions of health care (May, Durham and New 1980).

Payment for physician services was also affected by Nixon's Wage and Price Controls. Enacted in 1971, these controls limited physician and hospital fees and continued until 1976 (three years after other controls were lifted in 1973). Although U.S. physicians had themselves controlled fees in the past (through "fee bills" in the 1800s and informal regulation of local medical societies throughout the 20th century), this was the first time their fees were controlled by outside agencies and was indicative of the loss of autonomy of medicine that had developed since the 1960s.

It is clear that events regarding the payment for medical care are directly related to the issues of status and dominance that once again had come to the forefront in American orthodox medicine in the 1960s and 1970s. The rise of the federal government as a major third-party payer (and the ensuing regulation of those providing care to federal recipients), the rise of HMOs, PSROs and other measures to ensure the availability of care and cost-containment all reflected the diminishing status and dominance of medicine. These programs and policies also contributed to the continued diminishment of the status and dominance of medicine through the reduction of medicine's autonomy.

Funding of Medical Education Federal legislation regarding medical education altered the funding of this education and thus altered other important aspects of the social organization of medicine. In 1963 the Health Professions Educational Assistance Act involved the federal government in health education for the first time. This legislation, by linking financial assistance to the schools with increased enrollments, diminished the ability of medicine to control the supply of physicians (a crucial factor in the medical monopoly, according to Berlant (1975), since keeping the number of medical graduates low maximizes demand as well as prestige). The number of medical graduates almost doubled during the period under consideration here, rising from 6,994 in 1961 to 13,561 in 1976 (Campion 1984, p. 520). Amendments to the Health Professions Educational Assistance Act in 1965 provided for partial loan forgiveness for medical graduates who went on to practice in underserved areas, thus attempting to alter not just the number of practitioners but the location of their practice as well.

Changing Institutional Arrangements The institutional arrangements in the education of physicians and the practice of orthodox medicine began to change in the 1960s and 1970s. These changes had many ramifications for the unity of the profession as well as its status and dominance.

Health maintenance organizations (HMOs), which have existed since 1929, began to increase in numbers in the 1970s. In 1971 President Richard Nixon pushed HMOs as a key feature of his health care program for the nation and Congress passed legislation regulating and funding certain aspects of HMOs. HMOs come in a variety of forms: free-standing clinics, preferred provider arrangements, and so forth. Patients prepay their fees but payment methods to physicians vary. In all cases, however, the HMO set-up means there is an organizational layer that intercedes between physician and patient that reduces physician autonomy (Fielding 1984). Wolinsky and Marder (1985) note that both staff model HMOs and group model HMOs have lower levels of autonomy and more individual constraints than individual practice associations or solo fee-for-service practices.

Increasing medical specialization certification programs changed medical schools, hospitals, and the link between the two. In turn, these changes affected the medical profession. The number of full-time clinical faculty in medical schools increased by 214% between 1951 and 1960 (Powers, Whiting, and Opperman 1962). This represented a decrease in one of the few remaining institutional links between medical schools and physicians in private practice. As medical specialization gained momentum, the number of residents in graduate training programs increased (increasing 193% between 1951 and 1960 (Powers, Whiting, and Opperman 1962)). The link between medical schools and hospitals in metropolitan areas became stronger as hospitals came to rely more on house staff services provided by these residents and medical schools needed the hospitals to provide the clinical settings for these graduate programs.

The federal funding that began flowing to the medical schools for education and research in the early 1960s, the changing role of the medical school in the hospital system and the growing hospital system itself were all part of what Starr (1982, pp. 362-369) calls the new post-War structures of opportunity and power in medicine. The antecedents and consequences of these structural changes are numerous (see Kendall 1965; Miller 1977), but the basic phenomenon that is of interest here is the internal split in the profession of medicine between the growing numbers of physicians working in institutional settings and the relatively declining proportion of physicians in private practice. This structural division was central to the decreased unity of the orthodox medical profession in this period. Furthermore, the AMA, which was seen as representing the interests of the individual office-based practitioners, no longer represented the interests of the profession as a whole as the proportion of this type of practitioner decreased (as will be discussed shortly).

The changing position of hospitals in the health care system also had consequences for medical autonomy and control. The conflicts inherent in the "dual authority" hospital administration systems (Smith 1955) gained momentum in this period in light of several changes. First, the increased cost of medical care resulted in a push for efficiency in the provision of medical care and other cost containment considerations. This boosted the importance of hospital administrators. Second, as already noted, changes in third party payer systems, particularly the rise of the federal government as a major third party payer, placed administrators in a crucial position as hospitals strove to follow regulatory guidelines and optimize their position in the new health care system. Third, the increase in for-profit hospitals started in 1968 and these for-profits are typically characterized by a highly standardized and powerful central management (Starr 1982, pp. 430-436; Relman 1980) and decreased power and autonomy of the hospital's medical staff.

Changing Doctor-Patient Relations: The Rise of the Patient The 1960s and 1970s saw a number of significant changes in the relations between many physicians and patients. Generally speaking, these changes involved a relative increase in the status of patients and a relative decrease in the status of physicians. There were changes in the definitions of the patient's and physician's rights and obligations vis-a-vis one another. There were also changes that went beyond the actual doctor-patient encounter and involved changes in the definition of the entire context of that encounter, including expanding views of the health activities people are capable of (and even better at) doing themselves (so they need not *be* patients), and a questioning of the relative merits and detriments of many of the advanced technologies becoming available to patients during this time.

The growth of self-care, self-help groups and consumerism during this period were all part of these changing patient-physician relations (Schwartz and Siederman 1987). Self-care has always been the major form of health care in U.S. society. Schwartz and Siederman (1987) note that this form of health care may have started growing in the 1960s with the rise of religious groups emphasizing faith healing (such as the rise of Catholic Pentacostalism or the Charismatics in 1967). The burgeoning of the nonprescription medicine industry may also indicate this increased reliance on self-care.

Self-help groups of all types began to blossom in the 1960s and this trend apparently continues today (Schiller and Levin 1983). Alcoholics Anonymous, perhaps the quintessential self-help group, started in 1935 and many other self-help groups (as well as private professional therapeutic programs) have copied their approach of self-disclosure and mutual support. Withorn (1989) reports that health-oriented self-help groups have existed since the 1940s but really increased in numbers in the 1970s.

Another major impetus for self-help groups was the feminist health care movement which began in the 1960s and generated over 1,200 self-help health care groups by 1975 (Renzetti and Curran 1989). Self-help groups "frequently come to share vocal and strong criticisms of professionalism and professional care" (Withorn 1989, p. 419). Feminist health care groups in particular are typically very critical of the care given by professional medical practitioners. In the now classic *Our Bodies, Ourselves* (Boston Women's Health Book Collective 1973) women are counseled to take charge of their health care and are provided with information to assist them to that end.

Self care and self-help groups represent a clear challenge to the dominance of medicine in the medical arena and to the status of the physician in the doctor-patient relationship because they directly challenge the notion that the physician knows best (Savo 1983). This same challenge is posed more broadly by patients who seek medical care, according to Haug and Sussman (1969). These authors proposed that there was a "revolt of the client" beginning in the 1960s. This "revolt" consisted of the growing distrust of professionals and their abilities and the demand for client participation in medical decision making. Surveys from 1976 and 1979 investigating the patient's challenge to physicians' authority indicate that "[c]onsumerism in medicine is a reality in the United States" (Haug and Lavin 1983, p.181).

Historian John Burnham notes that the general status of the physician was beginning to decline by the 1960s. He says (1982, p. 1474):

During the first half of the 20th century, up until the late 1950s, American physicians enjoyed social esteem and prestige along with an admiration for their work that was unprecedented in any age.

This esteem declines in the 1960s and 1970s for a variety of reasons, says Burnham, including the social movements to promote lay control in medical decision making. But he also places this shift in a larger historical framework, arguing that the "entire society was moving toward social leveling" (1982, p. 1478) and had been moving in this direction almost since the turn of the century.

Organizational Setbacks in the AMA

The challenges to orthodox medicine's control over the provision of medical care in the 1960s and 1970s posed (and reflected) numerous problems for the medical profession in terms of its status, unity, and dominance. Changes taking place within the organization of the AMA, the leading professional association, also posed and reflected a set of problems for medicine in the 1960s. Most of the changes internal to the AMA resulted from changes occurring outside of the organization. Of particular importance were the loss of the Medicare-Medicaid battle, factionalism within the AMA, the changing organization of medicine, and financial and membership problems.

Defeat in the Medicare-Medicaid Battle It is difficult to overstate the impact of the loss of the Medicare-Medicaid battle on the AMA. AMA historian Campion (1984, p. 285) summarizes the effect as follows:

> No organization can undergo what the AMA did and remain the same. It had battled a generally hostile press, two Presidents of the United States and three Congresses - and lost. It had taken an uncompromising stand upon a major health issue, laid its principles on the line and committed its resources - only to fail.
>
> Outwardly the association appeared unscathed. No one was calling for resignation; no one was looking for a scapegoat. Nevertheless, feelings of disenchantment and unrest were running through the House of Delegates.

As I noted earlier, the AMA had vigorously opposed any national health insurance program for more than forty years and had pumped an enormous amount of its resources into the fight during the five years before the final defeat in 1965. This defeat represented a major loss to the AMA not only on the substantive issue at stake, but also in terms of its power and status as an organization. The AMA, in conjunction with state and local medical societies, had been successful at dictating U.S. health policy for almost a century. This dominance ended in the 1960s.

Factionalism within the AMA As I have noted before, the membership of the AMA has always had its share of differences. But the organization has also always tried to maintain a public front of consensus and unity and, more importantly, maintain a working consensus that allowed the organization to complete the business at hand. In the 1960s and 1970s, it appears that maintaining this working consensus was difficult indeed.

In 1965, with the Medicare and Medicaid legislation, AMA historian Campion (1984, p. 52) says "the factionalism reached peak temperatures." The Medicare-Medicaid issue was divisive in several different ways. First, there were those who dissented from the AMA's position opposing national health insurance or national health service. Physicians served on the Committee for Health Care through Social Security, which favored a compulsory national health system. Support for an expanded national health care system was higher among the academic physicians in the medical schools and among younger physicians in general. But the Medicare-Medicaid battle was divisive in another sense as well. There had long been debate between AMA "purists," as Campion (1984, p. 287) calls them, who saw the AMA as primarily a scientific association and those who saw the AMA as a political organization as well. This division was exacerbated during the 1960s when so many of the AMA's resources were being devoted to political ends. With the failure of the AMA's legislative efforts in 1965, the rift was in some ways deepened. The purists saw this defeat as an indication that the organization should not have been so involved in such legislative efforts in the first place and as fodder for their argument that the organization needed to stick to the realm of science and medical practice. Those who were politically-oriented saw the defeat as an indication that more resources and effort needed to be expended in the area of health politics (Campion 1984, pp. 285-299).

Factionalism within the AMA was not limited to disagreements over issues such as Medicare and Medicaid. As I noted earlier, there were numerous changes in the social organization of medicine (beginning in the 1950s) that affected the AMA of the 1960s and 1970s. For example, continued increases in specialization -- some with competing interests -- created very basic divisions within the membership. Changes in the institutional arrangements of the practice of medicine also affected factionalism within the AMA. The AMA had long opposed the corporate practice of medicine. Official opposition had been written into its code of ethics in 1912. Corporate medicine was opposed because it was seen as interfering in the doctor-patient relationship, creating a conflict of interest, and restricting the free selection of physician by the patient. When the hospital system began to expand, many physicians questioned whether there was a difference between practicing corporate medicine and practicing as a salaried physician in a hospital (Campion 1984, p. 189). In 1959, the AMA finally formally resolved this issue when a new policy was adopted by the House of Delegates that specified that patients be free to choose their doctor *or* to choose the health care plan they prefer. But the issue was not dead. As Campion (1984, p. 191) notes, "it would take several more years before many private, solo practitioners and county medical societies would stop looking at institutional medicine with a resentful eye." This was another instance of the factionalism that characterized the profession and the AMA as the decade of the 1960s began. As I noted earlier, the AMA had traditionally been dominated by the solo office-based practitioners. The changing social organization of medicine, with an increase in physicians working in organizational settings, meant that the traditional power base of the AMA was in decline and new power structures were to be forged.

Membership and Financial Difficulties Throughout the 1960s and 1970s the AMA faced a number of challenges that potentially threatened its very survival. Though none of these challenges proved fatal, together they created an organizational necessity to be on the defensive for almost two decades.

Membership losses through the 1960s and 1970s were a major concern for the AMA. By 1971, the AMA had only 50% membership (Starr 1983, p. 398). Starr says this decline is due to the fact that the AMA did not give sufficient consideration to "social changes." But also important was the revocation of unified membership requirements (that required members of state medical societies to join the AMA) in all but two states by the early 1970s (Campion 1984, p. 52).

Various financial difficulties plagued the AMA by the end of the 1960s and through the 1970s. One problem was the decline of advertising revenues generated by AMA publications. In part because of a slowdown in new drugs coming to market and in part because of competition in the medical advertising market posed by non-AMA publications, AMA advertising revenues declined by almost $3 million between 1967 and 1969. The AMA had 17% of the drug advertising market in 1960, 14.6% in 1967, and 7% in 1974. The AMA had a $3.3 million surplus in their budget in

1967. In 1969, the organization broke even. By 1970 it had an almost $3 million deficit and in 1971, after a membership dues increase, it still had a deficit of almost $1 million (Campion 1984, pp. 364-367).

Unity, Status and the Fight against Chiropractic

In chapter 3 I discussed the development of unity in medicine after the turn of the century and the importance of that unity, in organizational terms and in terms of collective identity and image. Unity again becomes an issue for the profession of medicine during this period of history from 1961 to 1976. Organizational unity is problematic due to the organizational setbacks in the AMA noted above. Unity of collective identity and image is an issue that relates to the perceived changing status and image of the AMA and the profession of medicine. The response of organized medicine to chiropractic is linked once again to these issues of unity and status.

Despite the many divisions within medicine in general and within organized medicine in particular during this period from 1961 to 1976, there appears to be agreement when it comes to collective pronouncements on chiropractic. For example, in JAMA chiropractic is increasingly referred to as a "cult" after the publication of the pamphlet "The Cult of Chiropractic" by the AMA in 1961. This is expanded to "unscientific cult" in 1966 after the publication of the pamphlet "Chiropractic: The Unscientific Cult." Indeed, the policy statement on chiropractic which is adopted by the AMA House of Delegates in 1966 -- itself an indication of the unity of opinion on this issue -- begins: "It is the position of the medical profession that chiropractic is an unscientific cult...."[58]

The unity of organized medicine's position on chiropractic is noted by the AFL-CIO's "Fact Sheet on Chiropractic" in 1970, which states:

> Though physicians are often divided on many issues, they are unified in their opposition to chiropractic theory and practice.[59]

Of course, there were some individual physicians who disagreed with this assessment of chiropractic.[60] But the public pronouncements indicate collective unity and I have never seen any indication of physicians collectively and publicly organizing in support of chiropractic.

As I indicated earlier, most of the items published about chiropractic during his period from 1961 to 1976 assume that there is consensus on this issue of chiropractic. The repetition of items that assume this unity serves to remind readers that this unity exists. The increased numbers and more prominent placement of items opposing chiropractic (in editorials and special articles) during this period indicates an upsurge in these reminders of unity. Beyond this, however, items published during this period appear to foster unity through the encouragement of unity of action against chiropractic. Many items include such calls for unified action:

> *All physicians* should urge their patients who have been victimized by cultists practices to make complaints to law enforcement officers.[61] (emphasis added)

> AMA's Department of Investigation has sounded an alert for *all physicians* to be on the lookout for chiropractors who attempt to gain hospital privileges.[62] (emphasis added)

> In fulfilling their obligation to protect the public health, *all physicians* have the duty now to call these pronouncements to the attention of the public.[63] (emphasis added)

> Therefore, I call upon *all* who share the responsibility of maintaining quality health care for the people of our country to give the people the facts about chiropractic.... [Y]ou will only be doing what you are obligated to do - protecting the public health.[64] (emphasis added)

> We believe it is vital that *every physician* should and must respond to the challenge [to exclude chiropractic services from Medicare].[65] (emphasis added)

These calls for unity of action against chiropractic are no doubt intended to have very concrete consequences (the demise of chiropractic or at least the continued exclusion of chiropractic from existing health institutions and financing mechanisms). But, in a Coser-like analysis of the positive functions of social conflict, these calls for unity of action also serve to remind physicians of their collective identity.

The activities of the AMA in regard to chiropractic and the materials that are published about chiropractic enable the medical profession to assert its professional claim to public service and dedication to the health and well-being of humanity. This is particularly important in this period of history in light of the accusations levied at the AMA by those who criticized the AMA's stance toward the Medicare-Medicaid legislation and those who supported increased consumer control over health care. These accusations included the charge that the AMA was self-serving and that physicians cared more about their incomes and control over health care than the health needs of their patients and the public. As noted earlier in this chapter -- and as evident in many of the quotations listed above -- opposition to chiropractic was couched in terms of orthodox medicine's dedication to protecting the public. This approach allowed orthodox medicine to reaffirm its commitment to public service and reassert its collective identity and image as a profession dedicated to such service. It allowed orthodox medicine to reassert its claim for professional status and prestige. As AMA Executive Vice President Dr. F.L.J. Blasingame noted in 1961:

> Needless to say, naivete toward chiropractic can lead only to increased public health hazards and inevitably, to lower esteem for the medical profession and all legitimate health sciences.[66]

Chiropractors frequently challenged this assertion and argued that medicine's opposition to chiropractic was self-serving not public serving. But medical publications denied such accusations and always recast the issue in terms of safeguarding public health. For example, a 1966 JAMA author states:

> Doctors of medicine oppose cultist practices, not because of any fear of competition, but from the desire to protect the public from the hazards of such practices.[67]

Another example comes from a response to a 1966 brochure published by the American Chiropractic Association:

> The confrontation between medicine and chiropractic is not a struggle between two "professions"; rather, it is in the nature of an effort by an informed group to protect the public from fraudulent health claims and practices.[68]

Issues of the status of medicine are implicit in the entire campaign against chiropractic. Stigmatizing chiropractic as "cultism" and "pseudoscience" is a way to indirectly advertise the superior scientific credentials of physicians. A more specific example of medicine asserting its own status as it denigrates the status of chiropractic can be found in the case of chiropractic education. Recall that in 1955 the AMA declined to investigate chiropractic education. By the early 1960s this inactive stance had changed and in 1964 the AMA published a special report on a 1963 study of chiropractic education that mimicked the investigations that were done in the 1910s and early 1920s. Seven letters of application were sent to chiropractic schools and the schools' response to these applications was noted. The letters came from fictitious persons, including a massage parlor operator, a truck driver, and an elevator operator. The report characterized the applications as "ludicrous," saying the applicants all had "inadequate educational, academic, and social backgrounds" and that the letters themselves were "ill prepared."[69] Most of the applicants were provisionally accepted, pending demonstration of high school equivalency. In 1966 the AMA Department of Investigation published a report "The Educational Background of Chiropractic School Faculties" which examined the college catalogues of thirteen chiropractic schools and concluded that the faculties were "inadequate."[70]

Discussion and Conclusion Early in the century, in the period from 1908 to 1924, there is a clear attempt to link the need for increased unity and status in the medical profession with the attempt to eliminate other healing practitioners, especially chiropractors. Such direct links -- made explicit by the medical profession itself -- do not appear in this later period from 1961 to 1976. I found no evidence of a conscious, intentional effort to target chiropractic as an issue around which physicians could rally and therefore "recapture" the organizational and occupational unity and status that had become problematic in the 1960s. Nor did I find evidence of any direct attempts to even link the idea of diminished unity or status with the efforts to oppose chiropractic. I argue, however, that the construction of such a direct link in the items that are published about chiropractic is not necessary.[71] The attention given to the opposition to chiropractic allows medicine to: 1) reaffirm its organizational unity on this issue; and 2) reaffirm its singular collective identity and image as superior professionals dedicated to public service. This happens whether medicine explicitly recognizes and acknowledges this link or not.

Medical Dominance and the Fight Against Chiropractic

The challenges to medical control over the provision of care that were posed by the federal government, by provider institutions and by patients themselves during the 1960s and 1970s, were challenges to the medical dominance that had been consolidated in the previous three decades. Why is it that organized medicine steps up its opposition to chiropractic just as it faces some of the most difficult internal and external challenges since the turn of the century? This action makes sense when one realizes that the opposition to chiropractic provided a mechanism through which medicine could attempt to reassert its dominance.

In its fight against Medicare and Medicaid, the AMA had stood in opposition to the American Public Health Association, the American Hospital Association, the American Nurses Association and many other health occupations and organizations. Through the battle against chiropractic, the AMA was once again able to align itself with these other health occupations and organizations. Chiropractic was characterized as the common enemy as many of these organizations ended up taking positions in opposition to chiropractic by the late 1960s and early 1970s.

The AMA initiated and led the fight against chiropractic. A 1969 JAMA editorial boasts:

> [U]ntil recently the effort to inform the people about the evils of chiropractic has been made almost exclusively by medicine.... That situation has now changed.[72]

The editorial goes on to list other organizations and recent legal decisions that now support the AMA's position.

As I noted earlier in this chapter, there are many items published in JAMA and AMN during this period that note the denunciation of chiropractors by various health groups and other organizations. The publication of these items may be seen as an effort to realign itself with these health organizations and take on a leadership role that demonstrates its scientific, social and ethical superiority. Orthodox medicine used the chiropractic issue to again assert its dominance in the medical arena.

The AMA also found itself in opposition to many nonhealth groups in its initial fight against Medicare and Medicaid, including the AFL-CIO and some senior citizens groups. When the AFL-CIO and the National Council of Senior Citizens came out with public positions supporting the AMA's position against the inclusion of chiropractic in federal health programs, this was given a great deal of coverage in JAMA and AMN.[73] Much coverage was also given to the 1969 HEW report "Independent Practitioners Under Medicare" that recommended that chiropractic not be included in Medicare.[74] This was significant because HEW and the AMA had "'less than cordial" relations during the battle over Medicare (Anderson 1985, p. 165). Likewise, attention was given to the report by the Task Force on Medicaid and Related Programs, which was composed of many nonphysicians and also recommended that chiropractic care be excluded from this federal program.[75] This extensive coverage contributed to the medical professions' efforts to reaffirm its dominant position as expert in all health-related matters, a position that had been challenged when these nonhealth organizations refused to support the AMA in the initial debates over Medicare and Medicaid.

Conclusion: Dominance The efforts to oppose chiropractic are not the result of any conscious or intentional effort to increase the dominance of medicine in the medical arena or in the eyes of the public. But the efforts of the AMA to *publicize* its stance against chiropractic do appear to be part of an intentional effort to assert a leadership position in the medical and public arenas on this issue. A 1964 JAMA editorial makes this clear:

> [P]hysicians have an obligation to promote the science and art of medicine and the betterment of public health. Notwithstanding their natural reluctance, physicians should be more aggressive educating the public as to the falsity of chiropractic claims.[76]

Through this highly publicized rhetoric and action against chiropractic, medicine attempted to reassert its dominance in the medical arena and in society.

Conclusion: Unity, Status, Dominance and Chiropractic as Enemy

Earlier in this chapter I characterized this final period of published medical reaction to chiropractic in terms of "chiropractic as enemy." I have argued here that this reaction can best be understood in the context of the problematic nature of medicine's unity, status, and dominance at this point in history.

I am not proposing a neat causal relationship between any single event that I have presented in this section and the reemergence of the battle against chiropractic. I am arguing instead that the entire constellation of events in the 1960s and continuing into the 1970s together threatened the unity, status and dominance of medicine and that this then was responsible for the resurgence of intense opposition to chiropractic during this period.

We can again explore certain alternative hypotheses. As I asserted earlier, the *scientific hypothesis* -- that orthodox medicine rejects chiropractic on scientific grounds -- is a constant that cannot explain the variations in the vigor with which opposition to chiropractic is pursued. The *medical competitor hypothesis* -- that variations in organized medicine's response to chiropractic can be explained by variations in the level of threat posed by chiropractic -- does not hold for this final period. For this hypothesis to provide adequate explanation, one would have to be able to demonstrate that chiropractic had indeed changed in ways that would pose an increased threat to orthodox medicine. There is some evidence, perhaps, that chiropractic gained strength near the end of this period (after 1972 or so),[77] but there is no evidence that chiropractic was an increased threat in 1961 when the campaign against chiropractic began or throughout the rest of the decade.

The *perceived medical competitor hypothesis* predicts that fluctuations in the response of orthodox medicine to chiropractic are due to perceptions on the part of organized medicine that chiropractic poses a threat to medicine. "Objective" changes in the status of chiropractic need not necessarily have occurred. In this hypothesis, medicine might increase the intensity of its opposition to chiropractic if it believes that chiropractic poses an increased threat. There is little evidence to support this view. Indeed, most medical publications report the state of chiropractic as pathetic, especially during the first ten years of this period. For example, a JAMA editorial reported the findings of a study in California:

> Chiropractic is not a "great, uncrowded profession," as chiropractic publications would have prospective students believe. Many of those in practice are doing so poorly that they have to supplement their income by other employment.[78]

This is certainly not perceived as threatening.

Medical Economics (ME) is the journal perhaps most likely to reveal any perception of any economic or other threat. Yet even here one does not see any such perception until almost 1974. A report in ME of the same California study mentioned above, entitled "Chiropractic is Cracking Up!", begins:

> Remember when chiropractic looked like a big threat to medicine? It may still be a sore spot on the corpus medicus; but according to a new study, it's fading fast.[79]

A special report in ME in 1968 proclaims in its title the "Beginning of the End for Medical Quacks," [80] although two months later there is an article about chiropractic being on the offensive to secure greater privileges.[81] But it is not really until 1974, with the publication of Vogl's article "It's Time to Take Chiropractors Seriously,"[82] that we see evidence of chiropractic being perceived as a threat. Although this is an interesting development, it does not contribute to our understanding of the battle against chiropractic that began in 1961.

As I noted at the beginning of this chapter, it is at first glance very surprising that organized medicine should spend so much time and energy writing about and actively opposing chiropractic during this very busy time in its history. In fact, some other AMA activities were temporarily limited during this period. For example, in late 1960 the AMA's Economic

Research Department reported that it was giving "less emphasis" to primary research so that it could spend more time on "the fight against legislation threatening the freedom of the private practitioner of medicine"[83] (referring, no doubt, to the Forand bill and the Kerr-Mills bill). And yet it is during this same period that the AMA is gearing up for its campaign against quackery in general (for example, planning for the 1961 National Congress on Medical Quackery, which it co-sponsored with the National Health Council) and chiropractic in particular (for example, starting on its pamphlet "The Cult of Chiropractic," released by the AMA Law Department in 1961). In the ensuing years medicine faced the King-Anderson bill, first introduced in 1961 and reintroduced over the next few years, along with the many other bills relating to health services for the elderly and other health matters. A great deal of organizational energy is nonetheless directed at chiropractic. This would be surprising if this battle against chiropractic -- or "public education program against chiropractors,"[84] as it was called -- was simply the public-serving activity that it claimed to be. It is much more understandable, however, from the perspective I have outlined in this chapter. For in fighting chiropractic, organized medicine is serving itself and the profession: focusing on unity in the face of factionalism, demonstrating its superiority in the face of a doubting public, and reasserting its dominance in the face of bureaucratic and legislative challenges to that dominance.

NOTES

1. JAMA Oct. 27, 1962, 182(4):407.
2. JAMA Sept. 19, 1966, 197(12):45 (notes that three of the second day presentations deal with chiropractic); JAMA Oct. 10, 1966, 198(2):10.
3. JAMA Oct. 24, 1966, 198(4):172.
4. JAMA Sept. 9, 1968, 205(11):10.
5. Bliss Halling, "Bureau of Investigation," in Fishbein (1947, pp.1034-1038).
6. Page 3 from *Chiropractic: The Unscientific Cult*. Chicago, Ill.: The American Medical Association, 1966 (23 pp.).
7. JAMA Nov. 23, 1964, 190(8):763-4.
8. JAMA Aug. 23, 1965, 193(8):10.
9. JAMA Oct. 24, 1966, 198(4):172.
10. JAMA Aug. 23, 1965, 193(8):10.
11. For example, it is noted that the *Did You Know That...?* pamphlet is available for $.05 for a single copy and $.01 each for 1000 copies (JAMA Jan. 31, 1966, 195(5):10). The *What They Say About Chiropractic* pamphlet is also promoted (JAMA Nov. 16, 1970, 214(7):1190; JAMA Jan. 25, 1971, 215(4):539-540).
12. JAMA July 25, 1966, 197(4):9.
13. JAMA Oct. 24, 1966, 198(4):172.

14. JAMA Apr. 17, 1967, 200(3):130.

15. JAMA July 29, 1968, 205(5):10.

16. JAMA June 16, 1962, 180(11):18.

17. JAMA Mar. 14, 1964, 187(12):15 ("Washington News").

18. JAMA Oct. 2, 1967, 202(1):46.

19. JAMA May 21, 1973, 224(8):1077.

20. JAMA Sept. 10, 1973, 225(11):1309.

21. JAMA Nov. 12, 1973, 226(7):722.

22. JAMA Oct. 24, 1966, 198(4):172.

23. For examples of items urging physicians to contact legislators regarding chiropractic see: JAMA Apr. 15, 1971, 216(1):147; JAMA Aug. 16, 1971, 217(7):959.

24. JAMA June 27, 1966, 196(13):249 ("Law and Medicine"). For other examples urging physicians to educate the public about chiropractic, see JAMA Mar. 14, 1962, 187(12):15 ("Washington News") and JAMA Nov. 23, 1964, 190(8):162 ("Editorial").

25. JAMA Oct. 26, 1963, 186(4):377.

26. JAMA Mar. 4, 1961, 175(9):833 (letter to the editor regarding Civil Air Patrol physical exams).

27. See footnote 11 above.

28. JAMA Jan. 25, 1971, 215(4):539-40.

29. JAMA Nov. 23, 1964, 190(8):162.

30. JAMA June 27, 1966, 196(13):250.

31. For examples of general calls for physicians to inform the public about the problem of chiropractic, see the following issues of JAMA: Apr. 14, 1969, 208(2):352; Sept. 15, 1969, 209(11):1712; Nov. 17, 1969, 210(7):1172; Richard S. Wilbur, M.D., "What the Health Care Consumer Should Know about Chiropractic," JAMA Feb. 22, 1971, 215(8):1309; and Mar. 12, 1973, 223(11):1210.

32. For items that report the rejection of chiropractic by radiologists, see the following issues: JAMA Mar. 31, 1962, 179(13):28; JAMA Sept. 22, 1969, 209(12):1800.

33. For items that report the rejection of chiropractic by the National Council of Senior Citizens, see the following issues of JAMA: July 7, 1969, 209(1):167; Nov. 17, 1969, 210(7):1172; Feb 22, 1971, 215(8):1309; Aug. 16, 1971, 217(7):959; Mar. 12, 1973, 223(11):1210.

34. JAMA Aug. 31, 1970, 213(9):1481-1482.

35. For items that report the rejection of chiropractic by the AFL-CIO, see the following issues of JAMA: Nov. 9, 1970, 214(6):1096; Feb. 22, 1971, 215(8):1308-1309; Aug. 16, 1971, 217(7):959; Mar. 12, 1973, 223(11):1210.

36. JAMA Sept. 11, 1972, 221(11):1296.

37. JAMA Jan. 14, 1974, 227(2):216.

38. JAMA Jan. 12, 1970, 211(2):183.

39. See the following issues of JAMA for coverage of the HEW report "Independent Practitioners Under Medicare": Mar. 17, 1969, 207(11):1991; Apr. 14, 1969, 208(2):352; June 9, 1969, 208(10):1971-2; Nov. 17, 1969, 210(7):1172; Aug. 31, 1970, 213(9):1481-2; Feb. 22, 1971, 215(8):1308; May 15, 1972, 220(7):1009;

May 21, 1973, 224(8):1077; July 8, 1974, 229(2):132.

40. JAMA Apr. 26, 1971, 216(4):586.

41. JAMA Sept, 15, 1969, 209(11):1712; JAMA Nov. 17, 1969, 210(7):1172.

42. JAMA Sept. 15, 1969, 209(11):1600.

43. JAMA Nov. 16, 1970, 214(7):1190.

44. JAMA Aug. 16, 1971, 217(7):959.   (Maisel's article is entitled "Should Chiropractors Be Paid with Your Tax Dollars?")

45. JAMA Feb. 11, 1974, 227(6):613.

46. *England vs Louisiana State Board of Medical Examiners* (246 F Supp 993). This case was given a great deal of attention. See the following JAMA issues: July 11, 1966, 197(2):20; Nov. 25, 1968, 206(9):2191-2; Apr. 14, 1969, 208(2):352; July 7, 1969, 209(1):168.

47. JAMA July 10, 1967, 201(2):162; JAMA Dec. 21, 1970, 214(12):2202. (These two articles are almost identical.)

48. JAMA Nov. 20, 1972, 222(8):1068; JAMA May 14, 1973, 224(7):1071-2.

49. JAMA Nov. 12, 1973, 226(7):829-30.

50. JAMA May 26, 1962, 180(8):35; appeal reported in JAMA July 21, 1962, 181(3):34.

51. JAMA Sept. 29, 1962, 181(13):31.

52. JAMA June 27, 1966, 196(13):249-50.

53. JAMA July 28, 1969, 209(4):487.

54. JAMA Dec. 1, 1969, 210(9):1816; June 22, 1970, 212(12):2177-8.

55. JAMA Aug. 31, 1970, 213(9):1481-2.

56. JAMA Aug. 16, 1971, 217(7):959.

57. JAMA Apr. 5, 1971, 216(1):147.

58. JAMA Apr. 17, 1967, 200(3):130.

59. As reprinted in JAMA Nov. 9, 1970, 214(6):1095.

60. Recall the *Medical Economics* survey in 1974 in which 5% of the physician respondents said they made referrals to chiropractors.

61. JAMA June 27, 1966, 196(13):250.

62. JAMA July 25, 1966, 197(4):9.

63. JAMA Apr. 14, 1969, 208(2):35.

64. JAMA Feb. 22, 1971, 215(8):1309.

65. JAMA Aug. 16, 1971, 217(7):959.

66. JAMA Oct. 21, 1961, 178(3):34.

67. JAMA June 27, 1966, 196(13):249.

68. JAMA Apr. 17, 1967, 200(3):132.

69. JAMA Nov. 23, 1964, 190(8):763-764.

70. JAMA Sept. 19, 1966, 197(12):169-175.

71. Furthermore, I think an argument can be made that the existence of such a direct link between the unity issue and opposition to chiropractic in the pages of JAMA and other medical publications would be surprising indeed.   There is much that differentiates the earlier period (1908 - 1924, where such a link was made) from this later period (1961 - 1976) that mitigates against the publication of such a direct link. In the later period, for example, there exists a more than forty-year editorial tradition, particularly in JAMA, of projecting an image of professional and organizational unity.

It is very rare for any issues of professional or organizational disunity to be noted in JAMA and the acknowledgement of such a unity problem in connection with the case of chiropractic would be very unlikely (even if it was recognized by AMA or other leaders).

72. JAMA April 14, 1969, 208(2):352.

73. See the following issues of JAMA for coverage of the National Council of Senior Citizens position on chiropractic: July 7, 1969, 209(1) 167; Nov. 17, 1969, 210(7):1172; Feb. 22, 1971, 215 8):1309; Aug. 16, 1971, 217(7):959; Mar. 12, 1973, 223 11):1210.

See the following issues of AMAN/AMN for coverage of the National Council of Senior Citizens position on chiropractic: July 31, 1967:1; Oct. 16, 1967:6; Jan. 20, 1969:4,9; Mar. 17, 1969:1; May 19, 1969:1,12; Nov. 10, 1969:10; Jan. 24, 1972:4; July 31, 1972:5.

See the following issues of JAMA for coverage of the AFL-CIO position on chiropractic: Nov. 9, 1970, 214(6):1096; Feb. 22, 1971, 215(8) 1308-1309; Aug. 16, 1971, 217(7):959; Mar. 12, 1973, 223(11) 1210.

See the following issues of AMN for coverage of the AFL-CIO's position on chiropractic: Mar. 16, 1970:10; Nov. 16, 1970:4; Jan. 24, 1972:4.

74. See the following issues of JAMA for coverage of the HEW report "Independent Practitioners Under Medicare": Mar 17, 1969, 207(11):1991; Apr. 14, 1969, 208(2):352; June 9, 1969, 208(10):1971-72; Nov. 17, 1969, 210(7):1172; Aug. 1, 1970, 213(9):1481-2; Feb. 22, 1971, 215(8):1308; May 15, 1972, 220 7 :1009; May 21, 1973, 224(8): 1077; July 8, 1974, 229 (2):132.

See the following issues of AMAN/AMN for coverage of the HEW report "Independent Practitioners Under Medicare": Jan. 13, 1969:1; Jan. 20, 1969:1,4; Jan. 20, 1969:4,9; Apr. 19, 1971:7.

75. See the following for coverage of the position on chiropractic taken by the Task Force on Medicaid and Related Programs: JAMA Aug. 31, 1970, 213(9):1481-2; JAMA Feb. 22, 1971, 215(8):1308; AMN Feb. 9, 1970:5.

76. JAMA Nov. 23, 1964, 190(8):772.

77. Possible evidence for an argument that chiropractic gained strength by the mid-1970s:

1. the last state to legalize the practice of chiropractic does so in 1974;

2. the Council on Chiropractic Education is designated the official accrediting agency by the U.S. Office of Education in 1974 (the first time an agency has been so designated);

3. chiropractic educational programs and research programs are strengthened (Wardwell 1982);

4. absolute numbers of people in the U.S. using chiropractic services increased from 4 million in 1966 (representing 2.3% of the civilian noninstitutionalized population)(US Department of Health, Education and Welfare [USDHEW] 1966) to 7.5 million (or 3.6% of the population) in 1974 (USDHEW 1978).

78. JAMA Aug. 6, 1960, 173(14):1582.

79. ME Aug. 14, 1961, 38:181.

80. ME Mar. 18, 1968, 45:23.

81. ME May 13, 1968, 45:98-107.

82. ME Dec. 9, 1974, 51:76-85.
83. JAMA Oct. 22, 1960, 174(8):1061.
84. JAMA Oct. 21, 1961, 178(3):34.

Chapter 6

Organized Medicine and Chiropractic Today: Unlikely Allies in Health Care Reform?

It was the fall of 1992 and for the citizen without health care insurance, it was exciting to hear presidential candidate Bill Clinton promise to bring universal health care coverage to the United States. For health care providers, however, this was a tension-filled time, for the call for health care reform could be answered in many ways. Not since the days of Truman had a president himself pushed so hard for health care reform. If Clinton were to win, no one was certain what form this reform would actually take. When Clinton did win, the uncertainty continued as he took many months to formulate and release an actual plan. The massive managed care arrangements that eventually emerged as key elements of the major 1994 health care proposals could have hurt any practitioners with solo and small group practices and a dependence on referrals. Chiropractors and physicians were not opponents in these reform efforts. Some medical specialists, chiropractors and other health care practitioners feared exclusion from the new health care systems and began to line up together against the idea of large managed care alliances. Other chiropractors hoped that the new emphasis on primary care would give them an advantage under any new system that emphasized a return to a reliance on such less expensive practitioners.

In the 1990s, with the push to reform a health care system that has become increasingly expensive, the relations between the professions of medicine and chiropractic are changing. The fact that chiropractors and physicians were present at some of the same hearings on the reform issues, that they testified before many of the same subcommittees, and that they proffered some of the same arguments and ideas is very significant. It was not that long ago, after all, that physicians were proscribed by their code of ethics from interacting in any manner with "cultists" (which included chiropractors). In part these changes are due to the mutual threat of managed care faced by elements within both of these groups. However, it is also clear that the changing relations between chiropractic and medicine cannot be completely accounted for by the economic pressures noted above. The social dynamics that played a role in the history of the relations between organized medicine and chiropractic must be considered in order to understand this latest twist in the tale. I argue that the changing alignment of chiropractic and medicine is due not just to external economic issues but to other changes within and outside each of these professional groups that cut to the core of their identities, status and power.

The health care reform efforts of chiropractic and medicine need to be placed in the context of the social changes within and outside each of these professional groups and their relative positions in the health care arena in the United States today. Chiropractic entered this most recent health care reform debate at its historical high point; there were more chiropractors than ever and never had so many chiropractic services been covered by third-party payers. Medicine, on the other hand, entered the health care reform debate at its historical low point; membership in the AMA was low and the administrative challenges to medical decision-making had been increasing dramatically.

During the months when the Clinton plan was being formulated, tensions ran high among health care providers, third party-payers and others who would be affected by the reforms. All the major players spent the ten months between Clinton's election and the release of the President's plan in September 1993 lobbying for their professional lives. The lobbying continued until health care reform efforts were abandoned in September 1994.

Although no health care reform package was passed by Congress in 1994, President Clinton and some members of Congress vow to raise the issues again. The rapid growth in the rate of health care costs has declined, but costs remain high and access to care continues to elude significant numbers of the population. This chapter will focus on the round of reform effort that fizzled out in the fall of 1994, but many of the issues continue to plague the country and the spark of reform may ignite once again.

CHIROPRACTIC INVOLVEMENT IN THE 1993-1994 NATIONAL HEALTH CARE REFORM EFFORTS

In November of 1992, the late Stanley Heard, who had been the Clinton family chiropractor in Arkansas since 1983, was asked by President-elect Clinton to define chiropractic for the new health care reform proposal that he would be developing. The Arkansas Chiropractic Association formed the National Chiropractic Health Care Advisory Committee (NCHCAC), with Heard as its chair. Members of NCHCAC included representatives from both the American Chiropractic Association (ACA) and the International Chiropractors Association (ICA) which made this effort an atypical collaborative endeavor.[1] The NCHCAC met with Clinton's Health Care Task Force and was asked to put together a position paper addressing: "managed competition, the economics of chiropractic in a national health-care system, chiropractic as a primary provider, and chiropractic as a gatekeeper."[2] On February 24, 1993 representatives from the ACA, ICA and the Association of Chiropractic Colleges met in Washington, D.C. and endorsed the NCHCAC as a joint venture.[3] The NCHCAC submitted its 223-page report, "Health Care for the 21st Century, Opportunities for Change: A Chiropractic Perspective," to Health Care Task Force Chair Hillary Rodham Clinton's office on March 23, 1993.

With the exception of this early joint effort, most of the rest of the health care reform activities of chiropractic appear to have been separately orchestrated by either the ACA or the ICA. Indeed on several occasions, the ACA was displeased with some of the activities of the ICA and vice versa. For example, on April 27, 1993, the student members of the ICA published a full-page "Open Letter to President Clinton and the White House Health-Care Task Force," which noted that studies by RAND Corporation and other organizations "continue to show the clinical effectiveness of chiropractic care."[4] Unfortunately, RAND took exception to this interpretation of its findings and notified the ICA and the ACA of this fact. The ACA then published in its journal a four-page series on this, publishing RAND researcher Paul Shekelle's comments and concerns about the misinterpretation of its findings as well as an editor's note about the errors in the ICA "Open Letter," comments by G. B. McClelland, President of the Foundation for Chiropractic Education and Research, and John J. Triano, Director of the Ergonomics and Joint Research Laboratory at National College of Chiropractic (each of whom emphasized the need to be scrupulously careful in discussing research findings), and a reprint of the report of the RAND findings which had originally been published in the *ACA Journal of Chiropractic* in 1992.[5] Nothing appeared in the *ICA International Review of Chiropractic* about the concerns of the RAND researcher.

Another incident occurred after the *Wall Street Journal* published a negative article about chiropractic by Timothy Smith in 1993. The ACA apparently responded to this article in what the ICA saw as a less than satisfactory way, and this, in conjunction with the disagreement above, may have been the end of any fragile coalition of these two associations. After the article was published, the ACA placed an advertisement responding to the article. This response condemned some of the chiropractic views and practices noted in the Smith article, gave support for immunizations, and in general, according to ICA critics, did not include enough negative information about the terrible safety record of orthodox medicine to counter the negative information about the safety record of chiropractic in the Smith piece.[6]

By the fall of 1993, there were still calls for unity of the profession in the health care reform movement but there was little evidence of joint effort. For example, at the ACA National Mobilization Conference in Dallas, where the ACA was announcing the details of Phase III and IV of its health care reform strategy before more than 100 chiropractic leaders, ACA President John Pammer stated:

> The ACA is carrying the ball for the entire profession. It is important that we communicate clearly on every level ... because only through cooperation and the unified efforts of all can we accomplish our objectives.[7]

The split between these two chiropractic associations plagued health care reform efforts just as it has plagued almost every other legislative effort on the part of chiropractic since the 1905 chiropractic practice act fiasco in Minnesota (where licensing was denied because straight chiropractors from Iowa came up to testify against the legislation) (Gibbons 1993). Mark Goodin, public relations consultant for the ACA, wrote a brutally frank report in January 1994 where he argued that unless chiropractors could come together and agree on the nature and scope of the profession there would be no chance for success at being included in whatever national health care reform takes place. Goodin basically expressed frustration at being placed in the uncomfortable position, when lobbying on behalf of chiropractic on Capitol Hill, of having to respond to questions like:

What about the other chiropractic professionals who seem to stray from that historical drugless, non-surgical foundation ... you know, those folks who are also licensed to provide nutritional supplements...? And just what is this business called chiropractic obstetrics and gynecology, and all this confusion about whether or not DCs are primary heath-care providers? Furthermore, what am I to make of those in the chiropractic profession who are providing care to animals, or adjustments under anesthesia? And what about this other culture which assigns an almost mystical and transcendental quality to vertebral subluxation?[8]

Clinton had demanded and received a single position paper, but after that the unity in the profession dissolved. Continuing the tradition of division which has characterized the profession for almost all of its one hundred years, the ACA and the ICA carried on parallel lobbying campaigns.

Chiropractic Health Care Reform Goals and Justifications

Even though the two professional associations could not work together for reform, they shared many of the same goals for this reform. After all, they defined the content or scope of their practices differently, but the structure of their practices was quite similar. There were three major features chiropractors wanted in any health care plan. First, they wanted the specific inclusion of chiropractic coverage in any mandated minimum benefits package. This could be either in the form of a specific mention of chiropractic or a "non-discrimination clause" that would specifically prohibit discrimination against non-MD providers in general and/or chiropractors in particular. Second, chiropractors wanted patients to be able to select particular practitioners. Chiropractors supported the "any willing provider" amendments regarding who could be included in a managed care plan and they supported having consumers choose whichever particular provider they wanted. This element was seen as particularly important, because it was feared that if chiropractic was included in a managed care plan that only allowed patients to see one or two chiropractors who are part of the plan, then most chiropractors would be hurt. Third, and finally, chiropractors wanted to have a gate-keeping role in any new health care plan. Chiropractors did not want physicians to be the gatekeepers controlling patient access to chiropractic care. In fact at one point, McAndrews argued that MDs should not be gatekeepers for spinal problems.

Chiropractors believed themselves to be in a strong position in arguing for their inclusion in any health reform plan. They noted, first of all, that chiropractic care features many of the very characteristics for which medicine had been criticized for lacking. Chiropractic focuses on prevention, is low-tech, and has a holistic orientation to the patient. (Some chiropractors added "drug-free" to this list.) Since the over-reliance on high-technology and lack of preventive care were two problems identified in the existing health care system and part of the reasoning behind health care reform in the first place, chiropractors saw this as a compelling argument in their favor. Second, chiropractic care is cost-effective care. Several recent studies showed spinal manipulation or specific chiropractic treatment to be cost effective in the treatment of back pain and chiropractors used this information to bolster their position. Since the high cost of health care treatment was one of the major factors behind health care reform, chiropractors argued this was a clear reason to support the inclusion of chiropractic care in any reform package. Third, chiropractors employed the "freedom of choice" argument that some physician groups were using as well, claiming that the American heritage of individual freedom dictates that consumers be allowed to choose who will provide their care. Lastly, chiropractors argued that the number of primary care providers is grossly inadequate and that chiropractic is in a good position to fill this gap in the health care system. Again, since the lack of primary care providers was also one of the major criticisms of the existing system, and had been for many years (with medicine allegedly doing little to remedy the situation), chiropractors believed this to be a strong argument in their favor.

ACA Lobbying Efforts

The January 1993 issue of the *ACA Journal of Chiropractic* dedicated eight full pages to "The Health Care Maze," a series of articles exploring health care reform and its possible implications for chiropractic. The articles in this issue outline the ACA's plan of action for making sure that chiropractic would be included in any national health care reform effort:

> It is an all-out effort, unprecedented in the history of chiropractic, to protect and guarantee the profession's future. Never before could one act of Congress make or break the profession, and never before has it been threatened with total exclusion.[9]

The original campaign plan had three phases: Phase I was educating DCs about the "nature of the threat;" Phase II was coordinating grass roots lobbying efforts; and Phase III would depend on the circumstances, including the success of the previous efforts, the money available, and the details of the final plan offered by Clinton. Sixteen specific plans were noted, including letter writing campaigns, television ads, one-on-one lobbying with members of Congress, coordinating efforts with state associations, and "[j]oint coalition efforts with other non-MD providers that share common concerns regarding health reform issues."[10]

Evident in these early days, too, were the calls for professional unity. For example, in January 1993 ACA Board Chairman Kerwin Winkler says:

> This is a time to put our petty family arguments aside and join together to get the job done for all, because a bad health-reform plan could affect the future of the entire profession.[11]

Chiropractic had a voice at the only public hearing before the President's Task Force on National Health Care Reform. R. Reeve Askew, of the ACA, testified at this 13-hour public hearing held on March 29, 1993 at George Washington University and moderated by Vice President Al Gore. There were a total of 66 panelists on 12 panels. Askew testified on the General Health Care Providers' panel as the only chiropractic representative (i.e., no ICA representatives). Other panelists represented: the American Nurses Association, the American Dental Association, the American Academy of Physician Assistants, the National Association of Social Workers, and the American Psychological Association. Askew gave a three minute opening statement (as did each of the others on the panel) and then engaged in a 45-minute question and answer period with Vice President Gore and the members of the Task Force.[12] Askew told the Task Force:

> Everyone agrees that expanded access to primary care is essential. However, the failure of medicine to provide an adequate supply of primary providers is well documented. In order to fill this gap, policies must focus on expanding access to non-MD providers such as chiropractors, nurse practitioners and others. Today, these providers are meeting the primary care needs of millions of Americans and have done so for years.[13]

Askew talked about the cost effectiveness of chiropractic in particular but emphasized the commonalities of chiropractic and other non-physician providers. He talked about the preventive orientation of the profession of chiropractic "and the other non-MD health professions" and said:

> I think the Task Force would be remiss if it did not take aggressive measures to ensure that Americans enjoyed expanded access to all primary care providers especially non-MD providers.[14]

Chiropractic also had a voice on the Health Professional Review Group

(HPRG), the group that reviewed the work of Hillary Clinton's Health Care Task Force prior to having the plan go to Congress. Chiropractor Jerilynn Kaibel, past president of the California Chiropractic Association, was appointed to this group as the sole representative of chiropractic (again, the ICA was not represented) and served on the HPRG with physicians, registered nurses, social workers, emergency medical technicians, pharmacists, a psychologist, physical therapist and other professionals. The HPRG met with Hillary Rodham Clinton, Chair of the Task Force, and Ira Magaziner, Director of the Task Force, for six days in April of 1993 and then again later in the year to comment on the final draft.[15]

On April 22, 1993 Jerome McAndrews, ACA Vice President for Professional Affairs, testified before the House Ways and Means Subcommittee on Health, chaired by Representative Pete Stark (D-CA) about being included in any minimum benefits package. McAndrews testified along with almost forty others, most of whom focused on the need for preventive care as a way to control costs, including representatives from the AMA, the American Optometric Association, the American Podiatric Medical Association, the American Physical Therapy Association, the American Hospital Association and the AIDS Action Council.[16] In his statement before the subcommittee McAndrews reviewed the ACA support for a comprehensive benefits package that supports:

> primary care, preventive care, and wellness.... In short, the benefits covered under national health reform should help steer our system away from high-tech, procedure intensive care toward holistic, preventive care. Otherwise, we build upon the current dysfunctional system which waits for illnesses to occur rather than one that attempts to prevent them.[17]

McAndrew then gave the utilization figures for chiropractic and noted that 85% of the insurance packages offered by employers currently cover chiropractic as do many federal health programs. He suggested that if chiropractic were excluded from the reform coverage it would be tantamount to reducing the care available and said "[w]e know of no policy maker who has suggested reforming the system by decreasing access to care"[18] (thus apparently trying to rhetorically cast the exclusion of chiropractic as being akin to the dreaded specter of rationing).

The ACA achieved most of its Phase I and II goals by the summer of 1993 and was awaiting the final release of the Clinton Plan so it could begin phase III (which included the plan to send out 45,000 copies of their analysis of the Clinton plan). The ACA summarized its activities to that point as follows:

The ACA and ACA-PAC are taking the national health reform issue seriously, investing well over a million dollars thus far in the Association's Emergency Mobilization Campaign, to fight for the future of the profession under national health reform. The funds have financed: the distribution of thousands of professionally prepared "lobbying kits" for DCs; thousands of specially produced video tapes to motivate and educate chiropractic patients; numerous legislative update and advisory bulletins; specialized research projects favorably comparing the qualifications and services of DCs with other health providers; the efforts of an expanded group of professional lobbyists on retainer to the ACA; special testimony and written materials for members of Congress; the coordination of local constituent meetings with targeted members of Congress; and the profession's first-ever campaign of nationally broadcast television ads.[19]

By the fall of 1993 the ACA had begun Phase III and IV of the Emergency Mobilization Campaign, which involved "profession-wide generic grass-roots campaigning, intensified grass-roots programs in key congressional districts and PR projects to support the government relations efforts."[20] These latter efforts included radio spots in the key congressional districts which were designed to "enhance the image of chiropractic as a solution to high health care costs and encourage listeners to write their member of Congress to insist on inclusion of chiropractic in the new health-care system."[21] They delivered all of the information on chiropractic effectiveness to Congress and the White House, including the recent *British Medical Journal* studies, the RAND report on spinal manipulation, and the Manga study (Canada).[22]

The ACA continued to keep members informed of the progress of the health care reform efforts. In January of 1994, they devoted the entire issue of the *ACA Journal of Chiropractic* to health care reform. They published the testimonies of Bruce Cladek (from the Health Care Financing Administration) and Raymond Scheppach (Executive Director of the National Governors' Association) before the House Subcommittee on Health and the Environment and of Donna Shalala (Secretary of the US Department of Health and Human Services) before the Senate Committee on Finance.[23] They offered readers a comparison of the health plans being considered in Congress.[24]

By February of 1994, when the ACA held its annual National Chiropractic Legislative Conference in Washington , D.C., the ACA-PAC acknowledged that it was the 4th largest of the health-related PACs and that it had received over $1.5 million in contributions. The conference itself was regarded as a great success, with over 500 chiropractors present. The attendees were addressed by ACA and ACA-PAC leaders as well as fourteen members of Congress, including Senator Orrin Hatch (R-UT), a long-time supporter of chiropractic, Senator Bob Dole (R-KS), Senator Tom Harkin (D-IA), Representative Richard Gephardt (D-MO), Representative Newt Gingrich (R-GA), Representative Bill Brewster (D-OR), Representative Edolphus Towns (D-NY) and others. Many of these members of congress expressed support for the inclusion of chiropractic under any health care plan adopted. For example, Hatch, who himself is an advocate for chiropractic, reported that Senator Ted Kennedy wanted chiropractic to be included in the reform package. Towns, who is a chiropractic patient and advocate, pleased chiropractors when he said "We need anti-discriminatory legislation that does not exclude health-care professionals [like chiropractic]."[25] Harkin, too, strongly endorsed non-discriminatory language saying:

> Some things are non-negotiable. Non-discrimination is non-negotiable. This [health care reform] should be consumer driven. The consumer ought to have a choice.[26]

Dole, too, supported chiropractic inclusion, saying in regard to health care reform, "We have got to get it right, and it's not right if you are not included."[27]

But not everyone at the conference supported the specific inclusion of chiropractic in health care legislation. Walter Zelman, Clinton senior policy analyst on health care reform, said that the Clinton plan specifically did not mention chiropractors because Clinton wanted the market to determine which plans are better. Zelman reported:

> Chiropractic is not mandated because we don't want to regulate how the alliances implement their health care plans.... The alliances will want to have plans that include chiropractic as a selling point.[28]

McAndrews, the ACA Vice President for Professional Affairs, had been scheduled again to testify before the Stark House Ways and Means Subcommittee on Health. He never got to testify, but the ACA published his prepared remarks later in the summer anyway and they encapsulated much of the effort by the ACA at this point in the campaign to aggressively argue for the place of chiropractic. There were no more general statements supportive of the inclusion of all non-MD providers; instead there were clear action statements that were directed to what by this time was the all-but-guaranteed emphasis on managed care in the health care proposals on the table:

> [C]hiropractors should be established as "gatekeepers" for low-back pain.

The management of low-back pain should be transferred from those medical physicians who are currently engaged in such treatment to doctors of chiropractic and the government will have to proactively insist on the above two actions in recognition that they will not take place without such assertive efforts.[29]

McAndrews also addressed other issues on the ACA legislative agenda -- such as increasing the chiropractic coverage under Medicare and Medicaid -- and urged members of Congress not to support the "watering down" of the antitrust laws[30] (apparently in reference to the AMA initiative to amend antitrust laws to make it easier for physicians to develop their own managed care arrangements).

ICA Lobbying Efforts

In January of 1993, the ICA began its health care reform efforts with ICA President R. James Gregg's "President's Message" column, titled "A Call to Arms - A Call to Reason." The call to arms was directed at ICA leaders and members and outlined the ICA plan to engage in "high-visibility" actions to make sure the new administration's policy makers and new members of Congress were aware of the importance of chiropractic. This plan included identifying 98 policy-making positions in the new government, a series of National Health Policy Forums, a chiropractic patient letter-writing campaign directed at the 98 policy makers, and a call to ICA members to engage in a variety of activities, including having each member recruit a new member. The call to reason was to be directed at the policy makers, urging them "to consider the wisdom of public policies that arbitrarily restrict patient choice of providers and compel beneficiaries to seek the care of expensive medical specialists because they are denied access to highly economical and cost effective care of the doctor of chiropractic."[31] The ICA-PAC began to solicit money especially for the health care reform campaign and a "political action kit" was developed which had model letters for patients to use in contacting legislators.

The ICA hired James Corman (a past member of the House of Representatives for 20 years) to be the chief ICA lobbyist in the House of Representatives and to be the Chief Legislative Counsel of the ICA. Corman had been active in promoting chiropractic during the 1970 debates over chiropractic inclusion in Medicare and Medicaid. Larry Meyers (of Meyers and Associates), who had previously worked in the Carter Administration and was legislative assistant to Senator Lloyd Bentsen, was hired to spearhead the Senate lobbying.[32] John White, who was active in Texas politics and then was former Chair of the Democratic National Committee, was hired to head the efforts to work with the White House on health care reform.[33]

As expected, the number one item on the ICA Legislative Agenda for 1993 was the "[i]nclusion of chiropractic services in any new federal program of health service delivery or federally-mandated insurance coverage."[34] Meyers, however, took an aggressive approach saying that now was the time to move on all of the items on the ICA federal legislative agenda. He argued that working on the other agenda items -- such as expanded coverage of chiropractic under Medicare and inclusion of chiropractic in the Civilian Health and Medical Program of the Uniformed Services (CHAMPUS) -- "will strengthen, not diminish the general effort to obtain inclusion in any national reform program."[35] Corman, too, was considering the lobbying efforts for health care reform as part of a bigger picture:

> With all national ears tuned in to the health care debate, serious media efforts to educate the public about chiropractic are bound to have extraordinary results. ICA is working hard to use this opportunity to both advance the status of chiropractic in the public policies of our nation and to enhance the public understanding of this valuable science.[36]

In April the student members of the ICA placed a full-page advertisement in the *Washington Post*, the "Open Letter to President Clinton and the White House Health Care Task Force" to which reference was made earlier. David Green, ICA Media Consultant, noted that this advertisement was responsible for two phone calls from the White House to the ICA.[37]

At the beginning of the fall of 1993, President Clinton's health care plan had still not been released although the signs were that it would be some type of managed-care plan. ICA President R. James Gregg told ICA members in his "President's Message" that theoretically this could work in favor of chiropractic -- since managed care plans aim to reduce costs and chiropractic is cost-effective care. He reminded readers, however, that "there are... too many lessons in the actual history of such plans to allow ICA to rely on cost-effectiveness alone to secure chiropractic's inclusion."[38] He continued:

> Managed care plans, like private insurance and many government programs, are just as likely to be dominated by medical bias as any other kind of program. Since the pool of resources is by definition limited, the struggle for those resources between professions is far more likely to heat up, not fall by the wayside on the basis of what is or is not the most cost-effective way to deal with a particular class of conditions.[39]

Like the ACA, the ICA feared a list of mandated services that would not include chiropractic, but also feared the "selected practitioner" approach of many managed care programs that would exclude all but a few chiropractors. The ICA clearly supported a reform package that included freedom of choice -- of chiropractic and of chiropractic practitioner.

After the Clinton plan was unveiled, ICA President R. James Gregg expressed concern that the proposal did not include guarantees that chiropractors would be included:

> Sure, the proposal authorizes and even encourages the utilization of non-MD providers. However, given the history of our profession, this is little comfort since even when we are written into the law, such as Medicare, someone in the bureaucracy always seems to be able to find a way to obstruct and impede chiropractic access.[40]

Gregg said the ICA would be introducing five amendments to the Clinton plan, addressing the changes quoted below:

A.   Revision of the benefits package to clearly mandate chiropractic services at all levels of the plan including HMO and PPO configurations.

B.   Specifying the definition of "primary health care provider" to include, at a physician level, the M.D., the D.O. **and the D.C.**

C.   Clarifying the gatekeeper role in managed care plans to eliminate the professional bias against chiropractic care.

D.   Strengthening and expanding the bill's anti-discriminatory language to include discrimination against any category of provider (D.C.'s, D.O.'s, M.D.'s, etc.).

E.   Reducing the scope of authority of the National Health Board. We are all well aware of what Congress passed relative to Medicare and what the bureaucrats have done to distort that intent.[41] (bold in the original)

James Corman summarized the ICA health care reform efforts in January of 1994, characterizing it as a "multi-dimensional" campaign that had included face-to-face lobbying, grass-roots communications, constituent group meetings and getting chiropractic's message out through the media.[42] The engagement of the media is seen as a particularly valuable strategy, because, as ICA Media Consultant David Green said, "[t]he media is the only way *you* can be assured that the chiropractic story will get through to legislators without interpretation, commentary or any kind of screening" (emphasis in the original).[43]

ICA members were provided with summaries of seven plans being considered in Congress as of the beginning of the year[44] (although not in as much detail as the reports in the *ACA Journal of Chiropractic*) and the ICA continued its own reform efforts. In July of 1994, for example, Life Chiropractic College West President Gerald Clum, who was an ICA board member, met with House Majority Leader Richard Gephardt (D-MO) and encouraged Gephardt to support "any willing provider" language and the specific mention and inclusion of chiropractic in any health care reform plan.

By the end of 1994, it was clear that a complete health care reform package was not going to be passed and with the "Republican sweep" of the elections, the outlook for reform in the near future was not bright. At this point the ICA quickly adopted a defensive stance to complement the offensive legislative agenda for the coming year. ICA President James Gregg expressed this defensive stance when he wrote about his fears regarding the new Republican Congress:

> Legislation that would override state insurance equality laws may find a favorable hearing in the new Congress, jeopardizing those critical protections such state laws afford chiropractor and chiropractic patient alike.[45]

With national health care reform off the table, the ICA leadership quickly focused on another potential threat to chiropractic.

INVOLVEMENT OF THE AMA AND OTHER MEDICAL GROUPS IN THE 1993-1994 HEALTH CARE REFORM EFFORTS

Unlike chiropractors, physicians as a whole did not have to worry about "regular medicine" being included in any health care reform plan. However, physicians were quite concerned about the structure of the delivery of that care. Furthermore, physicians, unlike chiropractors, already practiced in a wide variety of settings with different structural arrangements, so there was little chance that all physicians would agree on reform goals to the degree that chiropractors did. As you will recall from earlier discussions, most chiropractors have solo practices or practice in small groups whereas only 43% of physicians in 1991 practiced alone or with one other physician.[46] The proposals offered by physicians for health care reform -- and their reactions to others' proposals -- were varied depending on the types of medical practice and the structural arrangements of the care given by those physicians. Although the AMA had been opposed to virtually all health reform efforts of the past, the AMA supported reform efforts in the 1993-1994 health care reform efforts (Ayres 1996).

Medical Health Care Reform Goals and Justifications

The AMA had three primary goals for health care reform. First and foremost, the AMA argued for universal coverage. Universal coverage had been the official first-ranked goal of the AMA since 1989 and remained the first ranked goal until December of 1994, when the first round of the health care reform battle ended with no action. The AMA supported the employer mandate to provide this coverage until December 1993, at which point the AMA House of Delegates, under pressure from conservative members, voted to support either employer mandates or individual mandates or a combination of both.

Second, the AMA argued for patient choice of health plan, physician and other providers. Part of this argument was longstanding; the AMA had opposed what was called corporate medicine throughout the first half of this century and had argued for freedom of choice for patients for just as long. The call for patient choice for other providers was a new twist, and while the intent was no doubt to include the ancillary medical providers rather than chiropractors, the formal language of this goal simply specified "other providers." This element of the AMA legislative agenda was quite controversial. Specialists within the AMA (and the specialty professional associations) supported this requirement while the AMA members who practiced in managed care plans already -- as well as the HMO industry, of course -- opposed this requirement, saying it undercut their ability to manage costs.

The third major goal of the AMA for any health care reform was physician autonomy. This was primarily expressed in terms of a requirement for due process rights of physicians in managed care plans. The AMA particularly wanted a requirement that physicians could not be let out of a plan without a hearing and could not be let go from a plan because they were ordering too many tests, had too high a hospitalization rate or other reasons that related to quality of care. There were several other related items that physicians wanted, including: "enhanced self-regulatory powers;" a loosening of the anti-trust laws, particularly those that impeded physicians from organizing themselves into care plans; and caps on malpractice suits.

These goals were ultimately set forth in the AMA-designed and promoted Patient Protection Act, most of which ended up being introduced and supported by Senator Paul Wellstone (D-MN). In arguing for their legislative agenda, the AMA and specialist groups argued in terms of freedom of choice and in terms of the quality of care and level of expertise. Physicians in managed care spoke primarily in terms of their ability to stop the increasing costs of health care.

Medical Specialists versus Primary Care Providers

Sixty-four other medical groups signed on as agreeing with the AMA's legislative goals for health care reform. However, as noted above, there were several factions within medicine and these other medical groups and subgroups had other particular goals for health care reform. Some specialists' goals were to have gatekeeping privileges themselves. These specialists wanted to be considered primary care practitioners with direct access to patients. Dermatologists, for instance, were lobbying to be considered primary care physicians of the skin. Dermatologists had apparently already been particularly hard hit in HMO and other managed care plans because their expertise does not typically cover life threatening situations, making them an "expense " that can be safely cut. Dermatologists themselves have argued that most patients know when they need the services of a dermatologist, and so money can be saved by not requiring that the patient meet with a gatekeeper provider first.[47]

Some of these issues were already being negotiated at the state level. Medical specialists and nonphysician providers in several states pressed for legislation that would guarantee some direct patient access to their services in preferred provider organizations. For example, in 1994 Indiana apparently passed legislation that required some direct access to dermatologists and ophthalmologists (both MD specialists) as well as chiropractors and optometrists. Likewise, obstetricians-gynecologists (ob-gyns) have been successful in getting the gatekeeper status of the primary care designation. California provides a perfect example of this. In California, the issue of direct patient access to ob-gyns was framed as a women's rights issue, which no doubt played a role in the passage of this legislation. But the conflict surrounding the legislation also illustrates the divisions and shifting coalitions within medicine. The family practitioners in California, who otherwise could have been expected to oppose the designation of ob-gyns as primary care practitioners, entered into an agreement with the ob-gyns in December of 1993: the family practitioners would not oppose this change in ob-gyn status and, in return, the ob-gyns would not oppose the delivery of babies by family practitioners and would provide back up for these deliveries. Internists, however, did oppose the change in status of ob-gyns to primary care providers.[48]

There were several others reactions to the push to increase the number of primary care practitioners that played such a prominent role in the health reform debates. In June 1994, the AMA endorsed the development of guidelines specifying when primary care providers should refer patients to specialists. Such guidelines, they argued, should be jointly constructed by both specialists and primary care providers, fearing that unless organized medicine devised these guidelines they would be created by managed care administrators.[49] Retraining of specialists was also suggested by some as a way of meeting the need for generalists. Some places -- California and Boston, for example -- started offering relatively short retraining courses, but since these did not result in board certification (which has been a traditional way of evaluating physician competence in an area) it is not clear whether this type of training will be sufficient, especially to satisfy managed care administrators.[50]

Physicians in Managed Care

Another major faction within the medical profession was comprised of those physicians who already practiced in managed care settings. Some of these physicians actually lobbied against some of the elements of the AMA's Patient Protection Act, particularly those segments of the act that dealt with allowing patients to use providers outside the plan (which would defeat the cost-saving benefits of having specific and controlled providers).

Early in the summer 1994, the Group Health Association of America sponsored a massive effort to oppose the Patient Protection Act. Six-hundred HMO professionals, including physicians, lobbied congressional legislators to oppose this Act and to oppose all "any willing provider," "essential community provider," and "mandated point-of-service" proposals.[51]

AMA Reform Efforts

In January 1994 the AMA released their proposal for health care reform, the Physician Health Plans and Networks Act of 1994. They also launched an advertising campaign, including newspaper ads that asked the public who they want to trust with their lives: "an MD or an MBA?"[52]

On March 8, 1994, the AMA published a full-page advertisement in the *Wall Street Journal*, the *New York Times*, the *Washington Post*, and *USA Today*, featuring a letter to "Dear Senator/Representative." The letter, dated February 28, 1994, stated that the principles listed in the letter were agreed upon by each state medical society, by 64 medical specialty associations and by the AMA.[53] The letter featured the list of principles the AMA believed to be an essential part of any health care reform effort that were noted above:

universal coverage, provider choice for the consumer and physician autonomy.

In a speech to the AMA delegates in the June meeting in 1994, AMA Executive Vice President James S. Todd reported that AMA member physicians had distributed over a million brochures outlining the AMA health care reform plan. Additionally, the AMA had sent a letter to every physician and medical student (that is 740,000 letters) requesting them to ask members of Congress to support the AMA health care reform plan.[54] AMA organized a mass "house call" on Congress in early April of 1994, with more than 800 physicians descending on Congress to sell its plan and listen to the key congressional players who addressed the group (which they had done the previous year as well).[55]

PARALLELS IN MEDICAL AND CHIROPRACTIC HEALTH CARE REFORM EFFORTS

In reviewing the legislative goals, rhetoric and lobbying activities of chiropractors and physicians, several parallels emerge. In terms of the legislative goals sought by these two groups, three similarities appear. First, both MD specialists and chiropractors wanted a health care system that allowed for multiple gatekeepers. Neither group wanted access to their services determined by some single other gatekeeping group (such as general practitioner MDs). This goal was shared by other non-MD providers, such as optometrists and podiatrists, who also wanted direct access to patients. Second, both the AMA and chiropractors supported a requirement for patient choice, which would allow a patient to see any provider, even one outside of a plan. Third, the AMA and chiropractors supported "any willing provider" terms for determining which providers get to be in a particular managed care plan.

Both chiropractors and the AMA relied heavily on "freedom of choice" rhetoric to buttress their arguments. As was demonstrated earlier in this chapter, this powerful ideological link to culturally prominent conceptions of individual freedom was used over and over again by these health care provider lobbyists as well as by some legislators themselves.

ANY SIGNS OF THE EARLIER ANTI-CHIROPRACTIC EFFORTS IN THE CURRENT HEALTH CARE REFORM?

As you will recall from chapter 5, the last time the AMA was engaged in such a massive lobbying battle was during the 1960s when it was opposing Medicare and Medicaid legislation. At that time, it simultaneously launched the most concerted anti-chiropractic campaign in its history. In the current health care reform battle, however, the AMA said relatively little about chiropractic or any other non-MD provider groups. This is no doubt due at least in part to the legal constraints upon the AMA; since the *Wilk* case[56], where chiropractors successfully challenged the AMA and other medical groups as violating anti-trust laws, the AMA has published very little about chiropractic and virtually nothing that could be construed as trying to restrict the practice of chiropractic.

The only media campaign that addressed the issue of quackery and health care reform that received any publicity was an effort by the Texas Medical Association (TMA) that was not supported by the AMA.[57] The TMA produced a poster-sized brochure in order to raise funds for TEX-PAC and then sold the idea to eleven additional state medical societies. The brochure featured a large duck (actually, a goose) with large letters across the top saying: "Don't let reform duck up health care," with the subtitle reading: "Flocks of non-physician practitioner groups are using the call for health care reform as a decoy to lower licensing requirements and broaden their scopes of practice."[58] Another part of the brochure had the words "Quack, quack, quack" in large letters across the top of the brochure with the subtitle saying: "From Austin to Washington, non-physician health care groups are flocking to the forefront of the health care reform movement."[59] Jerome McAndrews, of the ACA, said he hoped to show these ads to members of Congress "to show the mentality that not just chiropractic is up against, but any alternate care.... I couldn't believe it when I saw that word [quack] again," referring to the penalties faced by physician groups in part for calling chiropractors quacks in the *Wilk v. AMA* anti-trust decision.[60]

DISCUSSION: HEALTH CARE REFORM LOBBYING AND PROFESSIONAL ISSUES

At the beginning of this chapter I stated that chiropractors and physician relations are currently being realigned and that the changing alignment of the two professions is due not just to the external economic pressures that were clearly posed in the alternative health care reform plans being considered. Rather, the issues that were raised during the months of health care reform activities -- and the changing alignments of chiropractic and medicine that were apparent in these reform activities -- are closely linked to other social changes within and outside each of these professional groups that cut to the core of their identities, status and power.

In this section I will first outline some of the changes that have affected organized medicine and the practice of medicine itself and then I will outline the very different effects some of these same changes have had on chiropractic. The gist of my argument here is that the social and organizational forces that have reduced medical dominance have actually benefitted chiropractic. The changes within the two professions are significant and have affected the relations between the two professions, both at the level of formal relations between the professional associations and at the level of individual practitioners. Distaste and distrust have not disappeared, but neither profession spent much time "bashing" the other in the public health care reform process.[61]

Changes in the Medical Profession and the Practice of Medicine: Implications for Professional Identity, Status and Power

Since the 1960s, the medical profession in the United States has experienced significant decline in its domination over the practice of medicine. As was detailed in chapter 5, challenges to medical control over the provision of care took place on several different fronts: payment for medical services, funding of medical education, changing institutional arrangements, and doctor-patient relations.

The federal government increased its role in the payment and provision of medical care. The 1960s spawned Medicare and Medicaid, Professional Standards Review Organizations, and the Comprehensive Health Planning Act. The 1970s saw federal wage and price controls that limited hospital and physician fees. The Health Professions Educational Assistance Act of 1963 diminished the ability of medicine to control the supply of physicians and also attempted to alter the location of their practice. The growth of HMO practice arrangements began to take off in the 1970s, with Nixon's support. The increases in medical specialization certification programs and the changes in the links between hospitals and medical schools were all part of what Starr (1982) called the new post-War structures of opportunity and power in medicine. Of interest here is the consequent split in the profession of medicine between physicians in institutional settings and physicians in private practice and the consequences the changing position of the hospital in the health care system had in terms of decreasing medical autonomy and control. The "revolt of the client" (Haug and Sussman 1969) and the increase in self-care were also part of the decline in medical domination.

The organizational structure of hospitals also changed rapidly during the last two decades, with the decline of community hospitals, the rise of the large hospital corporation and, importantly, with a decreasing role for physicians in hospital administration and management. In fact, delegates at the June 1994 AMA Annual Meeting approved a report stating that "the AHA [American Hospital Association] vision raises some major concerns for physicians.... [T]here is potential for hospitals to assume tremendous market power, threatening the clinical and economic autonomy of the physicians."[62]

These last few decades have also been a time of organizational setbacks for the AMA, beginning with the defeat in the battle over Medicare and Medicaid, as discussed in chapter 5. At the same time changes within medicine -- many of those noted above -- resulted in factionalism within the AMA and, ultimately a reduction in membership with corresponding financial difficulties.

The end result of these changes -- and the many other changes that I have not noted in this brief review -- was that organized medicine entered this latest round of national health care reform when it was at a historical low point. There was a great deal of factionalism within the AMA and AMA membership which, while almost 300,000, represented less than half of all physicians. AMA officials were, of course, aware of this and tried to call for unity and increased membership. For example, a January 1994 editorial in *American Medical News* (AMN), the politically and professionally oriented newsletter of the AMA, was titled "Professional Unity: Reform Stakes Too High to Risk Squabble" and stated:

A rent in the fabric of organized medicine is a problem for the profession at any time.... To begin unraveling medicine's strong professional unity now, midstream in the health system reform debate, is to court disaster.[63]

The specific complaint in this editorial was that the AAFP, the American College of Physicians, and the American Academy of Pediatrics had participated in a news conference where their representatives were standing on the stage with the Clintons to reaffirm their commitment to having an employer mandate as part of any health care reform plan (an idea abandoned by the AMA the month before).

There are many other examples of physician groups engaging in reform strategies independent of the AMA. The Association of American Physicians and Surgeons (AAPS), for example, sued the White House in 1993 in an attempt to force it to release the Task Force documents. Then in March 1994 it sued again, saying that the Task Force violated the Federal Advisory Committee Act of 1972. That law says that if a committee includes private citizens it must meet in public. Also, the AAPS charged the Task

Force with a conflict of interest, since members of the Task Force included participants with a major interest in the outcome of the health care reform efforts, such as the Kaiser Family Foundation and the Robert Wood Johnson Foundation.[64]

Likewise there are examples of the AMA joining with nonmedical groups to press their reform agenda. On July 20, 1994 the AMA issued a joint statement with the American Association of Retired Persons and the AFL-CIO, stating in part:

> Covering all Americans is essential to effective insurance reform, eliminating cost-shifting, and ensuring patient choice of physician and health plan... [This can be accomplished with a] shared employer-employee responsibility, with a required level of employer contributions.[65]

This alignment with these two more liberal consumer groups spurred House republicans, under the leadership of Representative Newt Gingrich, to send letters on August 1 to all AMA delegates as well as other medical association officials, charging that the joint statement displayed an endorsement of the Clinton/Gephardt health care plan and urging physicians to oppose the AMA position. In an August 4 meeting between AMA officials, Gingrich and Representative John Linders apparently resolved the confusion and the following week the AMA endorsed a House Bill based on the Rowland-Bilirakis bipartisan bill.[66]

In June 1994 AMA Executive Vice President James Todd warned physicians -- in a telling comment regarding the position of medicine in the health care reform debate -- that "if the profession wants to be considered a viable force in the future, it must not appear obstructionist."[67]

In August of 1994 an editorial appears in AMN that is uncannily like those pleas for AMA membership that occurred routinely at the turn of the century:

> Many physicians think they can do just fine without the AMA or a state society.... Yet everything points to a health care system that will be more complex, more arbitrary and - at the risk of sounding melodramatic - more hostile to physicians in the future. Rather than becoming less relevant, organized medicine will be needed more than ever before....[68]

Unlike the editorials of a hundred years ago, this editorial concludes by warning that physicians risk losing their voice if they abandon organized medicine. A hundred years ago they were trying to gain that voice. But if that happens, the editorial declares, using that phrase employed so often in those early editorials: "they'll have no one but themselves to blame."[69]

The fractured identity and decreased status and power of medicine resulted in organized medicine being just one more player in the health care reform process; it was no longer the dominant voice. At the December 1994 meeting of the AMA House of Delegates the association's legislative reform priorities were reordered, with the number one priority being "legislative protection of physicians and patient autonomy under managed care."[70]

This legislative focus is consistent with the current efforts by the AMA to provide support services for physicians regarding managed care, including consulting, education, workshops and even a new project to help find start-up funding for doctors who want to set up physician networks.

As the AMA increased its support of managed care it had to deal with the conflict between the specialists and the primary care providers among its ranks. AMA policy currently supports "point-of-service" plan options (required under the Patient Protection Act the AMA was pushing in Congress). Point-of-service options allow patients to see nonplan doctors. This satisfied the specialists, who otherwise are at the mercy of the primary care gatekeepers. But managed care plans opposed this, particularly the proposals that patients be allowed to select nonplan options without any higher costs and at any point (as opposed to just at the time of enrollment), saying it detracts from their ability to control costs.[71]

As part of the effort to recapture the unity and authority of the past, the AMA began rethinking its own organizational structure and its relationship with other medical associations. Additionally, a consortium of more than 160 medical organizations are evaluating their interrelationships. Says Robert Graham, head of the AAFP, of the search for a new organizational form:

> It's important to have a structure that would allow you to walk out after a major vote and tell the press and Congress that this represents the views of 80% of physicians in the country, rather than only the 40% that the AMA now represents. That would allow us to find a way to build in the voice of authority that we have lost.[72]

Changes in the Chiropractic Profession and the Practice of Chiropractic: Implications for Professional Identity, Status and Power

Many of the changes in the provision of medical care noted above were actually beneficial to the chiropractic profession. Changes in the payment for medical services tended to be a positive force for chiropractic. Chiropractic services were partially covered under Medicare and other government health programs and the inclusion of chiropractic services under private insurance plans increased. The increased role of government funding of medical education was a boon to chiropractic colleges and students who had historically been completely self-funded. The so-called rise of the patient probably had either a neutral or positive effect on chiropractic, which historically had always been client-centered and patient friendly.

The changing institutional arrangements that so radically altered the practice of medicine did not really affect chiropractic until recently. Since chiropractic practice was totally isolated from medical practice in the United States, the move to a more prominent role for hospitals, the rise of HMOs and managed care plans initially had no impact on chiropractic. As chiropractic began to become more of a "player" in the health care system, its interest in the shape that health care reform might take rose dramatically. The large managed care plans that were part of most of the health care plans on the legislative table had the ability to either bring chiropractic "into the fold" or exclude it completely. Although chiropractic survived "outside the fold" for decades -- and many have suggested that it survived *because* it was outside the fold -- many chiropractic leaders, particularly in the ACA, saw the exclusion of chiropractic from any national health care plan as potentially resulting in the end of the profession.

That chiropractic was such a prominent player in the health care reform process -- speaking relatively, of course (for example, AMA officials met with Ira Magaziner sixteen times, while there appear to be no instances of chiropractors meeting with Magaziner alone)-- is probably the result of the changes noted above, the result of the *Wilk* case, and a variety of other changes. A recent study found that many Americans are using alternative practitioners, including chiropractic (Eisenberg et al. 1993). Several studies have been published supporting the efficacy and cost-effectiveness of spinal manipulation in general and chiropractic in particular. Chiropractors are beginning to have expanded access to hospitals, particularly in terms of access to laboratories and imaging equipment.

Chiropractic remains a profession that is divided; it remains a profession of independent practitioners. Had a national health care plan passed, it may have had major consequences for chiropractic or it may have had almost none, depending on the features of the plan. At this point, chiropractic is back to seeking incremental expansion of the coverage of its services. Medicine appears only to be hoping to maintain what it has.

NOTES

1. In addition to Stanley Heard as Chair, the NCHCAC included: Gaylord Carter (Arkansas Chiropractic Association Legislative Chair) as Secretary-Treasurer; Sam Haley (ICA delegate from Arkansas) as Vice-Chair; Joe Balkman (ACA delegate from Arkansas); Gerald Clum (President, Association of Chiropractic Colleges); Arnold Cianciulli (ACA); John Hofmann (ICA); Rollie Dickinson (Congress of Chiropractic Associations); and Brad McKechnie (chiropractic consultant).

2. "Clinton Administration Gets Position Paper on Chiropractic," ("In the News" section), ACAJC June 1993, 30(6):78.

3. It is significant, however, that the ICA announcement of this meeting in its journal (which appears in a full-page advertisement-like format entitled "ICA Joins Profession-Wide Coalition on National Health Reform: Historic Meeting of Chiropractic Leaders in Washington, D.C." in the March/April 1993 issue of ICAIRC, 49(2):6) lists no ACA affiliations for any of the representatives attending this meeting. There is a list of representatives from chiropractic colleges which lists only the college affiliation (and ICA affiliation, if relevant) and a list of representatives from chiropractic organizations and associations which includes only ICA delegates and state association delegates. The ACA appears nowhere in this announcement, despite the fact that the text of the announcement emphasizes the profession-wide nature of this meeting:

> The meeting was the result of a strong desire with the profession for a united from at this critical time.... ICA whole-heartedly endorses the concept of a profession-wide effort and strongly supported the coalition that was born at this meeting.... (p. 6)

4. This "open letter" was reprinted in the May/June 1993 issue of the ICAIRC (49(3):6).

5. See "Misinterpretation of RAND Study Undermines Chiropractic's Credibility," ACAJC July 1993, 30(7):59-63.

6. The ICA journal published a piece by an independent public relations consultant who said the ACA ad was an unbelievably weak response to the *Wall Street Journal* article. See Stephen Tuttle, ICAIRC Sept./Oct. 1993, 49(5):12-13.

7. "ACA's National Mobilization Conference Draws Over 100 Chiropractic Leaders to Dallas," ACAJC Jan. 1994, 31(1):22-25, quoted on page 25.

8. Mark Goodin, "What's a Politician to Think? The Mantra of Primary Care and One Lobbyists Dilemma," ACAJC Jan. 1994, 31(1):19-21, quoted on p. 20.

9. "ACA Embarks on Emergency National Mobilization Campaign," ACAJC Jan. 1993, 30(1):26-29, quoted on p. 26.

10. *Ibid.* page 27.

11. *Ibid.* page 29.

12. "ACA Testifies Before Vice President Al Gore and Health Care Task Force," ACAJC July 1993, 30(7):101.

13. "R. Reeve Askew, DC, Testifies as Panel Member Before President's Health Care Task Force,"ACAJC May 1993, 30(5):71.

14. *Ibid.*

15. "Chiropractor Appointed to Clinton's Health Professional Review Group," ACAJC June 1993, 30(6):15.

16. "ACA Testifies Before Stark Health-Care Panel," ACAJC July 1993, 30(7):41, 101.

17. *Ibid.*, page 41.

18. *Ibid.*

19. "National Health-Care Reform: ACA Set to Launch Phase III of Emergency Mobilization Plan," ACAJC July 1993, 30(7):56-57.

20. "ACA Launches Mobilization Campaign, Phases III and IV," ACAJC Nov. 1993, 30(11):63-64, quoted on page 63.

21. *Ibid.*, page 64.

22. ACA Political Action Committee, "Common Questions and Answers About the Clinton Health-Care Reform Plan," ACAJC Jan. 1994, 31(1):27-30.

23. "Testimony Before the US House Subcommittee on Health and the Environment Regarding the States' Role in Health-Care Reform," ACAJC Jan. 1994, 31(1):31-37 and "Testimony from the Secretary of Health and Human Services Before the Senate Committee on Finance," ACAJC, Jan 1994, 31(1):39-45.

24. "A Comparison of Health-Care Reform Proposals," ACAJC Apr. 1994, 31(4):64-67.

25. Greg Lammert, "ACA's National Chiropractic Legislative Conference Draws Top Government Leaders," ACAJC Apr. 1994, 31(4):54-61, quoted on p. 59.

26. *Ibid.*, page 60.

27. *Ibid.*

28. *Ibid.*, page 61.

29. Jerome McAndrews, "Health-Care Reform's Impact on Managed Care," ACAJC July 1994, 31(7):32-34, 58-60, quoted on page 34.

30. *Ibid.*, page 59.

31. R. James Gregg, "President's Message: A Call to Arms - A Call to Reason", ICAIRC Jan./Feb. 1993, 49(1):7.

32. R. James Gregg, "President's Message: Responding to the Challenge," ICAIRC Mar./Apr. 1993, 49(2):7.

33. "The ICA Legislative Team," ICAIRC Mar./Apr. 1993, 49(2):9.

34. "Legislative Agenda," ICAIRC Mar./Apr. 1993, 49(2):10.

35. ICAIRC Mar./Apr. 1993, 49(2):13-14.

36. James. C. Corman, "President Clinton's Three Battles for Health Care Reform," ICAIRC Nov./Dec. 1993, 49(6):15-17, quoted on page 17.

37. David Green, "ICA/ICAPAC Media Campaign Takes Lobbying Effort to New Heights," ICAIRC Mar./Apr. 1994, 50(2):16-17, says this on page 17.

38. R. James Gregg, "President's Message: Health Reform, Managed Care and the Future of Chiropractic," ICAIRC Sept./Oct. 1993, 49(5):7-8, quoted on page 7.

39. *Ibid.*

40. R. James Gregg, "President's Message: What's Not in the Clinton Health Reform Bill," ICAIRC Nov./Dec. 1993, 49(6):9.

41. "Analysis of the Health Security Act of 1993 and the Outlook for the Chiropractic Profession," ICAIRC Nov./Dec. 1993, 49(6):11-13, quoted on page 13.

42. James Corman, "ICA Wages Multi-Dimensional Campaign to Protect Patient Rights and Promote Chiropractic in National Health Care Reform," ICAIRC Jan./Feb. 1994, 50(1):13-15.

43. David Green, "ICA/ICA-PAC Media Campaign Takes Lobbying Effort to New Heights," ICAIRC Mar./Apr. 1994, 50(2):16-17, quoted on page 16.

44. ICAIRC Jan./Feb. 1994, 50(1):15.

45. R. James Gregg, "President's Message: National Health Reform Revisited," ICAIRC Nov./Dec. 1994, 50(6): 9-10, quoted on page 9.

46. From *Medical Groups: A Comparative Analysis.* Chicago: American Medical Association, 1993, as reported in Mike Mitka, "AMA Study Says Group Practices Pay More, but Make Patients Wait," AMN March 7, 1994, 37(9):4.

47. Leigh Page, "Specialists as Generalists?" AMN Oct. 24/31, 1994, 37(40):3,38-39.

48. Leigh Page, "Specialists as Generalists?" AMN Oct. 24/31, 1994, 37(40):3,38-39.

49. *Ibid.*, page 39.

50. Leigh Page, "Retraining: On the Rise, but Are Specialists Interested?" AMN Oct. 24/31, 1994, 37(40):38.

51. Charles Culhane, "Insurance Industry Criticizes AMA Reform Bill," AMN July 4, 1994, 37(25):4.

52. Brian McCormick, "AMA Prescription: Give Physicians Greater Role, More Control Under Reformed System," AMN Feb. 7, 1994, 37(5):1, 25.

53. This advertisement was reprinted in AMN Apr. 11, 1994, 37(14):9.

54. "Dr. Todd: "H-Hour" for Health Care Reform," AMN July 4, 1994, 37(25):7.

55. Mary O'Connell, "Physicians Take Their Case to Congress," AMN March 28, 1994, 37(11):3, 20.

56. *Wilk et al. v. AMA et al.,* 1976. Complaint #76C3777 filed Oct. 12 in the United States District Court for the Northern District of Illinois, Eastern Division.

57. It must be noted that the Texas Medical Association (TMA) has the reputation for being particularly conservative. It was the TMA, for example, that lead the December 1993 move in the AMA House of Delegates to discontinue the AMA policy of supporting Clinton's employer mandate and instead have AMA policy support either an employer mandate or an individual mandate or both.

58. Julie Johnson, "Doctors' PAC Ads Outrage Other Providers," AMN Feb. 14, 1994, 37(6):7.

59. *Ibid.*

60. *Ibid.*

61. The ICA might be one possible exception to this statement, since some ICA pronouncements did include disparaging remarks about MDs, usually to the effect that medicine was intent on eliminating chiropractic and chiropractors.

62. Quoted in Janice Somerville, "AMA Warns that Hospitals' Reform Plan Could Hurt Doctor Autonomy," AMN July 4, 1994, 37(25):3.

63. AMN Jan. 10, 1994 37(2):17.

64. "Physician Group Charges Bias Among Reform Task Force," AMN Apr. 18, 1994, 37(15):4.

65. Quoted in Harris Meyer, "AMA Defends Reform Stand, Denies GOP 'Deal' Charge," AMN Aug. 8, 1994, 37(30):4.

66. Linda Oberman, "GOP Lobbies Doctors to Buck AMA Stance," AMN Aug. 22/29, 1994, 37(32):3, 7.

67. "Benefit of Membership," AMN June 13, 1994, 37(22):1. 11-12, quoted on page 11.

68. AMN Aug. 15, 1994, 37(31):15.

69. *Ibid.*

70. AMN Dec. 19, 1994, 37(47):1, 24, quoted from page 1.

71. "AMA to Help Members Cope with Managed Care," AMN Dec. 19, 1994, 37(47):1, 22.

72. Linda Oberman, "New Foundation? AMA, Federation Seek a Stronger Structure," AMN Nov. 28, 1994, 37(44):5.

Chapter 7

Professional Control and the Social Construction of Deviance

Earlier chapters depict the concrete processes through which organized medicine attempted to define and label chiropractic and chiropractic practitioners as deviant throughout this century. Although organized medicine was consistently negative in its stance toward chiropractic, as we have seen, the vigor of this opposition varied across time.

The "social construction of reality" perspective (Berger and Luckmann 1966) has provided the basic framework for the conceptualization of the analysis thus far. While this perspective offers us a most important insight into the nature of the phenomena under consideration -- that definitions of reality are socially constructed and are therefore manipulable -- theorizing in this perspective has typically been limited in focus to the process of reality construction. Most analysts have stopped short of placing this process in the broader context of other societal processes and structures. I have tried to push my analysis further in this direction. What accounts for the variations in the efforts of organized medicine to construe chiropractic as deviant? And why focus attention on chiropractic in particular? In this chapter I will attempt to answer these questions in the context of sociological research in the fields of deviance and occupations.

You will remember that the efforts of organized medicine to construct reality -- including the definition and labeling of chiropractic as quackery -- are part and parcel of their attempt to increase their own status. I suggested that their status was not an isolated issue but was instead part of the effort to maintain their occupational integrity, to maintain the boundaries of their group. Thus if we want to account for the timing and targets of their reality construction efforts (who gets labeled and when), we must look at what is happening to and within the medical profession in general and organized medicine in particular. In addressing these questions of timing and target I hope to shed light on how the definition of others as deviant is basic to the process of professionalization.

WHY CONSTRUCT DEVIANTS?

The sociological answer to this query begins with Durkheim's analysis of the necessity of deviance. As one of the early voices of sociological functionalism, Durkheim (1962) argued that deviance was necessary in any society. Durkheim thought deviance was necessary in society for two contradictory purposes (Ben-Yehuda 1985): 1) to promote the integration of society by clarifying its moral boundaries; and 2) to promote the flexibility of society that will enable it to successfully adapt and therefore survive.

Erikson extends Durkheim's analysis of the necessity of deviance. In his book *Wayward Puritans* (1966) he demonstrates that the definition of Antinomians, Quakers, and witches as deviants in the Massachusetts Bay Colony was a function of the need for increased solidarity in that community. When the community was threatened, deviants were created and caste out, thereby restoring the group's moral boundaries. Erikson's analysis does not account for the particular targets in this deviance construction process; indeed, he suggests that the group was reaffirming their solidarity in a general sense, not reacting to the nature of a particular act per se.

Also stressing the necessity of deviance in society, Ben-Yehuda (1985) argues along Durkheimian lines that the construction of deviance is central to both the processes of social stability and social change. For example, he notes that deviant sciences function to promote flexibility and change through the extension of scientific knowledge, citing the initially deviant but later accepted theories of continental drift and radio astronomy. Deviant sciences also function to promote stability, he says, through the solidarity-reinforcing process of resistance to such deviant sciences.

Adding the element of power to this discussion, Gusfield (1963) places the construction of deviants in the framework of status competition. He argues that when a group perceives another group as a threat to its own viability or dominance, it may attempt to stigmatize the other group in an effort to maintain its own position. He thus analyzes Prohibition in the

United States as an attempt by the native, rural, protestant middle-class to symbolically assert their domination over the growing and increasingly powerful urban, immigrant, Catholic lower-classes.

Inverarity (1976,1980) argues that the Durkheimian assertion regarding the necessity of deviance has actually been subject to little in the way of empirical testing.   Inverarity argues that sociologists must begin "distinguishing in general terms those kinds of social systems to which it is applicable from those to which it is not.... If Durkheim's proposition is not to be applied in an ad hoc manner, the general conditions under which it holds must be specified in advance" (1980, pp. 198-199). He notes that although some research supports the notion that societies will create deviance as part of the process of maintaining solidarity, this research is limited to smaller, pre-industrial societies characterized by mechanical solidarity. Current research actually provides little in the way of support for Durkheim's proposition when applied to modern, highly-differentiated societies characterized by organic solidarity.

Perhaps because he focuses on the issue of repressive versus restitutive forms of justice and the cult of the individual, Inverarity ends up ignoring the thrust of his earlier arguments and so ignores the substantial literature available on the group basis of modern society. I think that it is reasonable to assume, for example, that Durkheim's proposition would operate at the group level. Thus even if one was studying the construction of deviants in a modern, differentiated society, one could assume that the deviance construction processes that Durkheim analyzes on the societal level might take place on the group level within any particular society. Gusfield's analysis of prohibition and Lauderdale's (1976) experiments with the creation of deviance in small groups certainly suggest that this is the case.

I argue that Durkheim's analysis of the necessity of deviance can be (and has been) fruitfully applied at the group level. Group reaction to deviance can function to integrate groups and maintain group boundaries just as societal reaction integrates society and maintains societal boundaries.

TIMING

If we accept that group reaction to deviance functions as part of group efforts to integrate and maintain boundaries, we must still ask what accounts for this reaction at particular points in time. It is not enough to say that the reaction to deviance takes place when deviance occurs, since I have argued that deviance is a constructed phenomena, one that exists only in the context of reaction. In general, what accounts for the construction of deviants at particular points in time? In particular, what accounts for the efforts of organized medicine to construct chiropractic as deviant and for the variations in these efforts at different points in history?

In examining the literature in deviance, most analysts point to the existence of a strain or threat to account for the construction of deviants, for it is this strain or threat that accounts for the need to reaffirm group identity and increase solidarity. Durkheim (1947, p. 459) points to strain when he says "when a society is going through circumstances which sadden, perplex or irritate it, it exercises a pressure over its members, to make them bear witness, by significant acts, to their sorrow, perplexity or anger." Erikson (1966, p. 68), too, discusses the timing of the reaction to deviance in terms of the threat or strain experienced by the society: "The occasion which triggers this boundary crisis may take several forms - a realignment of power within the group, for example, or the appearance of new adversaries outside it...."

In his discussion of deviance, Ben-Yehuda (1985) argues that societies are more likely to construct deviance during times of transition. Periods of transition strain the existing definitions of reality (which support existing structures of authority) and therefore increase the need for reaffirmation of group identity and solidarity.

The case of organized medicine and its construction of chiropractic as deviant provides an excellent illustration of this process. The intensity with which chiropractic is opposed is clearly a function of the strains associated with the rise of medical dominance at the beginning of the century and the efforts to retain this dominance when challenged later in the century. It is easy to see this as a case of transition engendering the construction of deviants.

Ben-Yehuda's proposition that deviance is more likely to be constructed during times of transition is clearly an advancement in the more general propositions of Durkheim and Erikson. An integration of Ben-Yehuda and Erikson results in the following proposition: that the boundary crises that constitute the threat to the society (or the group) and spur the creation of deviants occur during times of societal transition. But such a proposition needs to be further refined, particularly if we are to meet Inverarity's challenge to the relevance of the original Durkheimian formulation in modern, highly-differentiated societies. After all, in such societies it appears that transition -- and strain -- is more a constant than episodic occurrence. And if strain is a constant, of course, it cannot be a factor explaining the timing of varying deviance construction.

The nature of the transition that engenders the construction of deviants needs to be further specified. In his discussion of the witchcraze in Europe during the 15th, 16th, and 17th centuries, Ben-Yehuda argues that the major strain was the "differentiation process" (1985, p. 58) involving the commercial, demographic and urban changes of this period and the demise of the Church's authority. In contrast, in examining the development of orthodox medicine in the United States in the 20th century I am focusing on a particular group within a society rather than society as a whole, within a much shorter time frame, and under conditions of rather continual change in an already highly-differentiated society. What can be learned about the dimensions of transition that appear to be relevant to the promotion of the construction of deviance from this case?

Orthodox medicine obviously underwent tremendous changes across the 20th century. Many of these changes involved new medical diagnostic and treatment techniques (such as technical changes and the introduction of new drugs), but the variations in the construction of chiropractic do not correspond with the introduction of such changes. Rather, as was shown in earlier chapters, the variations in the intensity with which chiropractic is opposed occur when the unity, status and occupational control of orthodox medicine is threatened.

At this point it is necessary to turn from the theoretical work in the field of deviance to the theoretical work in the field of occupations. As was noted in chapter 1, an occupational group seeks recognition as a "profession" because there are concrete benefits for an occupation so labeled (Becker 1962). Throughout most of the twentieth century, the primary benefits for professions are occupational autonomy and control.[1] A profession is considered to be an autonomous occupation, one that is able to control the content of its work and the conditions under which its members labor. This autonomy and control means that the profession assumes a dominant position in the structure of the relationships it has with other occupations (Freidson 1970, 1971). In order to secure this autonomy and control, occupations must be legitimated by relevant publics and the state. Securing this legitimation, in turn, requires unity and status. Professional associations work on behalf of their members to obtain legal legitimation; to be effective, such organizations require unity or at least an appearance of unity or a working consensus. Legitimation also requires a relatively high level of occupational status (in the sense of social esteem), although this is somewhat more circular in its effect (high status means greater likelihood of securing state legitimation, but state legitimation brings higher status).

Autonomy and control are thus central to the profession, for this is what distinguishes them from other types of occupations and defines them as a profession. To link this back to the social construction of deviance, I suggest that periods of transition that relate to professional autonomy and control would be the type of transition that would potentially strike most centrally at an occupational group (whether they be transitions potentially increasing or decreasing that control and autonomy).

The social construction of chiropractic as deviant by orthodox medicine supports this idea. At the turn of the century and through the early 1920s, orthodox medicine was seeking to secure the professional prize of autonomy and control. It attempted to secure state and public legitimation and required unity and status to do so. As I demonstrated earlier, the outraged opposition to chiropractic was an integral element in this process of professional development, for it was a mechanism through which organized medicine could foster unity, assert its superior status, and secure for itself professional dominance.

When orthodox medicine's occupational control was potentially threatened by the suggestions and proposals of various health committees, conferences and the proposed federal legislation in the late 1930s and early 40s, the efforts to stigmatize chiropractic were temporarily intensified. When orthodox medicine's occupational control was potentially threatened in the 1960s and 1970s -- and ultimately somewhat successfully challenged -- the efforts to define chiropractic as deviant soared again.

TARGET

In addition to accounting for the timing of deviance-defining activities, an explanation is needed to account for the targets of these activities. In general, what accounts for the selection of certain groups or categories to be defined as deviant? In particular, why does organized medicine focus attention on chiropractic?[2]

Sociological research and theory in the field of deviance offers some guidance in this area but there are no clear answers. On the one hand, Erikson (1966) extended the Durkheimian analysis of the functions of deviance by suggesting that the particular activity which becomes the focal point for deviance-defining efforts is not really important. On the other hand, critics, such as Chambliss (1976), argued that Erikson reached that erroneous conclusion because he had ignored the benefits that elites accrue when particular groups or activities are targeted as deviant. For example, from a conflict perspective, outlawing the use of opium by the Chinese in California in the late 1800s (Lowes 1966) provided potential concrete benefits to the non-Chinese workers who believed that the Chinese posed a threat to their own work opportunities. Likewise, Gusfield (1963) argues that rural native middle-class Protestants supported Prohibition because they thus received the symbolic benefits of demonstrating their dominant status over the urban immigrant lower-class Catholics for whom alcohol was culturally important.

Turning to the case of the efforts of organized medicine to define chiropractors as deviant, neither the Eriksonian functionalist nor the conflict approach alone seems satisfactory. To suggest that organized medicine targeted chiropractic for no reason at all seems questionable on the face of it. But it is equally difficult to argue that organized medicine would have derived any clear benefit from having successfully opposed chiropractors in particular. Chiropractors never posed a serious threat to the survival of orthodox medicine or to its quest for dominance. Even if organized medicine had been successful in eliminating chiropractic, it is not clear that there would have been any resultant concrete benefits for medicine (although, of course, there no doubt would have been symbolic benefits).

However, focusing on chiropractic as a target for deviance-defining activities did allow organized medicine to accomplish certain desired goals. In the early years of this century (1908 to 1924) the rhetoric about the need for fighting cultists in general and chiropractic in particular was an important element in the push for organizational unity (which then enabled medicine to successfully pursue professional dominance).

Selecting chiropractic as a target provided certain advantages for organized medicine in this regard compared to other possible targets. There were no established interoccupational relations between chiropractic and orthodox medicine which could have posed difficulties for medicine. Such difficulties were faced by organized medicine as it fought the nostrum industry (Burrow 1963), for example, since medical practitioners had relations with both the more legitimate and less legitimate producers and distributors of such medicines and since some medical publications derived income from nostrum advertising. With chiropractors as the target, there was no complicating factor of religious freedom, as was the case with opposition to Christian Scientists. There were no chances that internal divisions within medicine would be brought to the forefront with chiropractic as the target. That could have been a problem with the fight against antivivisectionists because that was a more central issue for medical educators and researchers (and the increasing status of those groups was already creating some resistance among traditional general practitioners who wanted to make sure that the art of medicine did not become totally subordinate to the science of medicine).

In the early years of this century, orthodox medicine was also involved in an attempt to increase its social standing. Chiropractic provided a foil against which medicine could favorably compare itself (chiropractic practitioners being portrayed as uneducated members of the lower- or working-class). This made chiropractic a desirable target. Christian Science was started by the apparently well-educated and respectable Mary Eddy Baker who established a church in 1882 in Boston and attracted well-educated and well-situated believers (Reed 1932). Christian Science could thus not provide the social class nor general educational contrasts that chiropractic could. Homeopaths were also fairly well-educated and by this time were beginning to be absorbed within the ranks of orthodox medicine (Kett 1968). There were other types of healing practitioners at this time in history that were uneducated or had a lowly class background, but it appears that none of these were large enough enterprises -- or as geographically dispersed -- to be singled out as a unifying target as was chiropractic.

In sum, in the period from 1908 to 1924 orthodox medicine was pursuing the unity and status that it believed would enable it to achieve professional dominance. The most useful target for the deviance-defining activities that were part of this process would be a target that could enable medicine to promote its unity and status. Chiropractic was such a target.

In the period from 1961 to 1976 there is again a surge in organized medicine's deviance-defining activities and there is again a link between the issues of unity, status and dominance and the targeting of chiropractic as deviant. As discussed in chapter 6, this period follows an increase in the structural differentiation of orthodox medicine as well as increased factionalism within organized medicine. Unity is reasserted through the campaign against chiropractic, for "all" agree to the opposition of chiropractic.[3] To the extent that medicine perceives its status to be questioned by those promoting self care and consumer control over medical decision making, chiropractic again provided a good foil for medicine to use to demonstrate its own superior status and expertise. Fighting chiropractic "for the public good" allowed organized medicine to counter those alleging that medicine in the U.S. had become too self-serving.

CONCLUSION

Ben-Yehuda's (1985) proposal that societies are most likely to engage in the social construction of deviants during times of transition is an important refinement of Durkheim's (1962) original proposition regarding the functions of deviance and Erikson's (1966) expansion of this proposition. In a modern complex society, however, transition may be more a constant than episodic phenomenon. The type of transition needs to be further specified. Applying this theoretical framework to the deviance construction activities of an occupational group within modern society and combining it with the concepts of occupational control and professional dominance allows one to conclude that the timing and targets of these deviance-defining activities can be accounted for by the particular type of transition: change that involves occupational dominance.

NOTES

1. It is important to remember, as Johnson (1972), Larkin (1983) and Freidson (1986) point out, that the conceptualization of profession -- for both social scientists and lay persons -- has been rooted in a particular historical period. The active interpretations of what it means to be a profession and the structural possibilities that accompany this occupational status are themselves related and are related to other aspects of the social historical context.

2. Organized medicine may have focused their deviance defining activities on other groups or activities as well. Certainly there is editorial ridicule of other groups such as antivivisectionists and Christian Scientists in the pages of JAMA. However, I have no systematic evidence in this regard.

3. Surely there were those in the AMA who questioned the use of valuable time and money to fight chiropractic. But these objections were not made public in JAMA or AMN. There were very few items published earlier in the century that indicated any questioning of the efforts to oppose chiropractic (e.g., JAMA April 25, 1931, 96(17):1409-1410). I place "all" in quotation marks to remind the reader that this is a socially constructed "all" that does not necessarily mean "100%."

Chapter 8

Conclusion

It has now been one-hundred years since chiropractic began in the small town of Davenport, Iowa. Davenport, like many river communities, has changed tremendously in that time period: from its development into a booming river town through the decline of the river as the industrial and agricultural lifeline and now to the rebirth of the town that has come with riverboat gambling. Throughout this period, chiropractic in Davenport -- embodied in the Palmer College of Chiropractic -- has also had its ups and downs, although its residence at 1000 Brady Street has provided a stable presence on the hill leading up from the river for almost a century. The changes within the chiropractic profession have been no less startling than those in the town of Davenport. The distance from the hapless chiropractor being jailed for practicing medicine without a license to the chiropractic health care professional reporting to the President regarding its place in a new health care system is far indeed.

How has this happened? How has chiropractic managed to survive, thrive even, to celebrate its 100-year anniversary? Ironically, the answer to that question is probably wrapped up in the opposition of orthodox medicine to chiropractic. Walter Wardwell argues compellingly that chiropractic survived in large part because of the unity and determination generated by fighting organized medicine. Says Wardwell (1992, p. 178):

> The AMA attacks created in chiropractors and their supporters a sense of

righteous indignation at being persecuted.... Although the division between straights and mixers gave organized medicine leverage in legislative contests, chiropractors never lost sight of who their real enemy was.

But the focus of this book has been organized medicine, not chiropractic. I have argued that organized medicine's efforts to define chiropractic as deviant were not a direct response to the competitive threat posed by chiropractic. Rather, I have argued that these efforts represented a response the orthodox medicine's own varying quest for unity, status and dominance throughout this century. This adds a new dimension to the existing scholarship regarding the relations between chiropractic and organized medicine, most of which has focused on or at least implicitly assumed competition as the central dynamic in these relations (with competition conceptualized in economic or market terms) (e.g., Wardwell 1982; Coburn and Biggs 1986; Anderson 1981; Cobb 1977). Indeed, this emphasis on competition has been part of many studies of alternative or limited healing professions or practices, such as the analyses of optometry (Begun and Lippincott 1980), osteopathy (Albrecht and Levy 1982); midwifery (Wertz and Wertz 1977; Ruzek 1980), and homeopathy (Kaufman 1971). Competition has been accorded a central role in many analyses of the development of medicine as well (e.g. Berlant 1975; Feldstein 1977; Kronus 1976). By applying an analytical framework from the sociological study of deviance, I have tried to look at the issue of the relations between organized medicine and chiropractic in a way that moves beyond the concept of competition.

MOVING BEYOND COMPETITION: THE SOCIOLOGY OF MEDICINE AND CHIROPRACTIC

As is evident in the title of his article, "Chiropractors: Challengers to Medical Domination," Walter Wardwell (1982) examines how chiropractors have represented a threat and a challenge to medical domination across their history. The article includes several interesting arguments regarding the survival of chiropractic. But Wardwell starts with the assumption that orthodox practitioners dominate the medical arena, that chiropractors challenge that dominance, and that orthodox medicine responds by fighting chiropractic. My analysis indicates that this is not quite the case. Rather, orthodox medicine begins the 20th century *in the process of* attaining dominance and that its early opposition to chiropractic is a central part of this process. Medicine's opposition to chiropractic is not consistent across the century and the variations can be accounted for not so much by what chiropractors are doing (as "challengers") but by developments in the social organization of medicine itself.

Wardwell has studied chiropractors themselves and this vantage has yielded many important insights for the sociology of chiropractic in particular and the sociology of medicine in general. But different insights can be gleaned by switching vantage points and studying orthodox medicine's opposition to chiropractic.

David Coburn and C. Lesley Biggs (1986) have also provided an excellent history and analysis of the survival of chiropractic, although their study examines the Canadian experience. They argue, as I have, that the development of medicine and chiropractic must be placed in the context of "the dynamics of the society of which they are a part" (1986, p. 1037). While orthodox medicine's reaction to chiropractic is not their primary interest, Coburn and Biggs basically assume that medical opposition to chiropractic in Canada has been unvarying across this century (or at least until the 1970s). In the course of arguing that both the decline of medicine and the rise of chiropractic have been influenced by the increased role of the state in health care in Canada, they point to the reasons why organized medicine is no longer so concerned with chiropractic (1986, p. 1045):

First, chiropractic is no longer a prime danger or competitor for patients. Although it is true that recently medicine has been showing signs of being overcrowded, it is also the case that medical insurance guaranteed payment for all physician services.

Second, medicine as an organized group has a bigger fight on its hands. With state involvement in health insurance medicine sees itself directly threatened, chiropractic is less of a direct concern to the majority of the profession, particularly as chiropractic, as we have shown, has tended to narrow its scope of practice to one not challenging to the medical profession as a whole.

This is a version of what I have called the *medical competitor hypothesis* and, as I have shown, this type of analysis does not account for the variations in opposition to chiropractic in the United States. In fact, as far as the most recent period of history is concerned, I found that rather than abandoning their concern with chiropractic when they had the "bigger fight" of government involvement with health insurance to contend with, organized medicine in the United States *intensified* their opposition to chiropractic. Given that the conditions of medicine, health programs, the state and other features of Canadian society differ from those in the United States (Marmor

1982), it is possible that organized medicine in Canada simply responded differently to chiropractic. But Coburn and Biggs did not systematically measure the response of organized medicine to chiropractic across the years of their study and the empirical basis for the summary remarks I quoted above is not clear.

Like Wardwell, Coburn and Biggs have studied the issue of medical dominance and chiropractors using chiropractors as the focal point. One of their primary questions is how chiropractic survived in the face of medical opposition. Like Wardwell, they view chiropractic primarily as a challenger to medical dominance. In fact, Coburn and Biggs treat the survival and rise of chiropractic as an indicator of the decline of medical dominance that began in the early 1960s in Canada. In the work of both Wardwell and Coburn and Biggs, medical opposition to chiropractic is assumed rather than examined. These authors assume that chiropractic is perceived and responded to as a threat. The analysis in this book shows that the process is not that simple. While the perception of chiropractic as a threat to medical dominance may account for some portion of medicine's opposition to chiropractic, it does not account for all of it. For when this issue is studied using medicine as the focal point, it is apparent that the intensity of medicine's opposition to chiropractic has fluctuated over time and that these fluctuations are due not to any increase or decrease in the challenge posed by chiropractic. Rather, the intensity of opposition to chiropractic has fluctuated in response to the social development of orthodox medicine itself.

MEDICINE'S OPPOSITION TO CHIROPRACTIC: IMPLICATIONS FOR THE STUDY OF DEVIANCE

This book is a continuation of the research tradition established by Erikson with his work *Wayward Puritans* (1966) and continued by Ben-Yehuda in *Deviance and Moral Boundaries* (1985). As I noted in chapter 7, I have attempted to add greater specificity to the understanding of the timing and targets of deviance construction activities.

There is one other significant difference between my work in the area of organized medicine and chiropractic and the studies of deviantization by Erikson and Ben-Yehuda. Both of these authors have focused on groups that have experienced a "loss" of some type or are what one could call societies in decline. The definition of deviance is always discussed in relation to the reaction to this loss or decline. For example, Erikson analyzes the persecution of the Quakers in the Massachusetts Bay Colony in terms of the loss of elite status that was the result of increasing religious tolerance. Ben-

Yehuda analyzes the European witchcraze in terms of transition, but the focal points of this transition are the decline of the Catholic Church's dominance and the general end of the feudal order. Gusfield (1963), too, analyzed the creation of deviance (during Prohibition) that went along with the decreasing status of a previously dominant group in U.S. society.

Ben-Yehuda (1985, p. 71) goes so far as to say that the creation of deviance is part and parcel of the end of a community:

> Generally speaking, it appears, then that when a community so vehemently and desperately tries to restore its moral boundaries, it is doomed to fail. It is possible that the very attempt is in itself a symptom that profound change is taking place, that it is impossible "go back," so to speak. In this sense, the persecutions can be interpreted as symbols of incapacity, of a system's failure, as "death throes," if you wish, and they might be viable proof that the previous equilibrium cannot be recaptured.

In the case of organized medicine it is clear that the deviantization of chiropractic in the U.S., particularly in the early stage from 1908 to 1924, was not part of the demise of anything but was part of a beginning -- the "rise of the sovereign profession," as Starr phrases it. Orthodox medicine was certainly not in its "death throes," though it was very much involved in establishing boundaries. Thus my research indicates the often implicit assumption that the creation of deviance is associated with groups and societies in decline must be reexamined.

MEDICINE'S OPPOSITION TO CHIROPRACTIC: IMPLICATIONS FOR THE STUDY OF PROFESSIONS

This research contributes to the study of professions by demonstrating how the deviantization of one occupation can be an integral element in the professionalization of another. The idea that the deviantization of one occupational group by another can be a mechanism through which the professional prize is sought is a new element in existing models of professional development. Furthermore, this research shows how the process of professional development is grounded in particular historical circumstances -- including the definition of profession. As these circumstances change, so, too, do the deviantization efforts of the occupation.

FUTURE RESEARCH

The present research raises some interesting issues and questions for those interested in the process of the development of professions and deviance. A fruitful exploration of the timing and target issues in the construction of deviance could be pursued by comparing the deviantization of chiropractic with organized medicine's response to other alternative healing groups. Are there variations in the levels of opposition to these other healing occupations? Does the timing correspond to the variations in opposition to chiropractic or are there differences? Does the content of the deviantization relate to the timing? Here I would suggest comparing organized medicine's response to a limited scope occupation, such as optometry, and another broad scope alternative, such as Christian Science, in order to see whether and how this affects the response.

It would be worthwhile to investigate the efforts of organized medicine to oppose chiropractic in a smaller arena, such as a state-level study or even an analysis particular cities or counties. This would allow for a more thorough evaluation of the medical competitor hypothesis in relation to the deviantization of chiropractic. Although I have argued that chiropractic never really constituted a competitive threat on the national level (nor was it perceived as such), on the state or local level this might have been different. One possibility would be to compare the medical response to chiropractic in states that had a high chiropractor to physician ratio with the response in those states with low ratios. Reed (1932, p. 132) notes that some states, like Iowa and South Dakota, had a 1 to 4 D.C. to M.D. ratio whereas Virginia had a 1 to 86 ratio and Massachusetts had a 1 to 26 ratio. States could also be compared based on their chiropractor to population ratio (see Wardwell (1982, p. 233) for these variations). A state-level analysis would also allow for greater study of the role of the law in the processes of deviantization of chiropractic and the establishment of professional dominance (in accordance with Freidson's (1986) suggestions).

CONCLUSION

I do not wish to fall into the trap of historical functionalism by suggesting that the changing requirements of the medical profession across this century *demanded* the particular responses to chiropractic that were observed, a trap which Abrams (1982, p. 113) calls "the worst kind of a-historical historicism." I have tried to retain an emphasis on the specific historical context, in terms of how profession was defined, in terms of the changing

social structures of medicine and society, and in terms of the role of human agency in the interpretation of that context and the deviantization of chiropractic.
As Weber says in *The Methodology of the Social Sciences* (1949, p. 72):

> We wish to understand on the one hand the relationships and the cultural significance of individual events in their contemporary manifestation and on the other the causes of their being historically *so* and not *otherwise*. (emphasis in the original)

I have attempted to be true to the concerns with chiropractic that were created by and consumed orthodox medicine across this century, but I have also tried to look at why these concerns were "so and not otherwise."

Appendix A

Methodological Appendix

This study was basically an inductive enterprise. Although I had certain preconceptions about the relationship between organized medicine and chiropractic, those preconceptions had little to do with the path this study eventually followed. I began the study thinking I would document the consistent opposition of organized medicine to chiropractic. The opposition turned out to be variable. I began by thinking an examination of medical journals would provide clues to the activity of organized medicine vis-a-vis chiropractic. I ended up realizing that the materials in these publications were important in their own right, as the rhetoric and accounts that constitute the deviantization of chiropractic. I write this appendix on the research methodology of this study having already completed the analysis. The issues that I address are the issues I now see as being central to the study and to the defense of the study. I did not necessarily see these at the outset.

This is a study of the relationship between the process of deviantization, which is the process of socially defining an entity as deviant, and the development of occupational control. In particular, it is a study of the process through which organized medicine attempted to define chiropractic as quackery during the years 1908 to 1976 and how this related to medicine's attempt to achieve and maintain professional dominance during these years.

Deviantization is a public process. Defining another group as deviant must be done out in the open -- not necessarily before the public at large but certainly in front of the relevant audience or audiences. In this case, since I am analyzing how the deviantization of chiropractic was part of the process through which organized medicine developed and attempted to retain professional dominance, the most important audience consists of physicians themselves. The general American public and the state and federal legislatures are audiences of only secondary importance. My data therefore consists primarily of communications written by and directed at physicians.

THE DATA

The data for this project includes all materials that are published about chiropractic in the *Journal of the American Medical Association* (JAMA), *The New England Journal of Medicine* (entitled *The Boston Medical and Surgical Journal* until 1928), and *Medical Economics*. These articles were analyzed in terms of frequency, form and substance. The indices for articles on chiropractic in *American Medical News* (entitled *AMA News* until 1969) were analyzed. Numerous other materials were also used, such as histories of medicine, histories of the AMA, histories of chiropractic, and pamphlets and other materials regarding chiropractic that were published by medical organizations.

Analysis begins in the year 1908 with the first mention of chiropractic in JAMA. The end point for the analysis is 1976, the year that chiropractors filed an antitrust suit against the AMA and other medical organizations and the point at which these organizations then stopped publishing materials opposing chiropractic.[1] The study continues by looking at the current health care debate, but this is a separate analysis, since materials about chiropractic were no longer being consistently published by organized medicine after 1976. Instead, for the analysis of the participation of organized medicine and chiropractic in the current health debate I primarily relied upon materials published in JAMA, *American Medical News*, the *ACA Journal of Chiropractic* and the *ICA International Review of Chiropractic*.

Primary Data Sources

JAMA is the major primary data source for material on the deviantization of chiropractic by organized medicine. This is the major data source for several reasons: 1) it is the major publication of the most dominant and inclusive medical organization in the United States; 2) it has the largest circulation of all medical publications in the United States; and 3) it has been published consistently across the entire period under study.

The JAMA data includes everything ever written about chiropractic in the pages of JAMA. This material was located in several ways. The manner in which items were indexed changed over the eight decades examined in this study. Accordingly, slightly different procedures were used to locate items on chiropractic in different time periods. In the early years, before chiropractic appeared as a separate category in the JAMA index, I searched through all materials under the following Index headings: Chiropractic, Christian Science, Osteopathy, Lay Medicine, Antivivisectionists, Fraud, Quackery, Medical, Politics, Profession, Irregulars, Iowa Medical News, and Editorials and Medicolegal (when these categories were listed separately, as of 1900). After 1901, the index was also searched under the headings AMA and Medical Practice, Organization, and Legislation. The items under these listings were then scanned for any mention of chiropractic. In 1908 chiropractic was first listed as a category in the JAMA Index. From 1911 to about 1952 chiropractic was listed consistently in the Index and the following listings in the Index were scanned: Chiropractic, Medicolegal (not published after 1959), Medical Practice Acts, and Malpractice. During most of this period any item published in JAMA that had the slightest reference to chiropractic was listed in the Index under Chiropractic. After 1952, the listings under Chiropractic decrease. At least part of this decrease appears to be a change in indexing procedures or policy (possibly related to the retirement of Morris Fishbein as editor of JAMA). In order to maintain as much consistency as possible in reporting the number of chiropractic items published each year, all articles were searched under the following additional Index categories after 1952: Cult, Quack, Manipulation, AMA, and Department of Investigation. After 1970 items listed under the category Health Occupations were also scanned. In this manner about one item per year was located that referred to chiropractic but was not listed in the index (and would have been listed under Chiropractic in earlier years).

The Boston Medical and Surgical Journal (BMSJ), which changed its title to The New England Journal of Medicine (NEJM) in 1928, was another primary data source for this project. I did not rely upon BMSJ/NEJM as heavily as I did JAMA for a number of reasons. First, it is published by the Massachusetts Medical Society and, particularly in the earlier years, there is more regional organizational coverage. Second, BMSJ/NEJM published relatively few items concerning chiropractic before 1920 or after the 1930s. I initially wanted to examine the materials on chiropractic in BMSJ/NEJM because although it is a regional publication, it is a prestigious medical journal with a large national circulation and it has been published continuously across the eight decades covered in this study. In the end I used the data from BMSJ/NEJM as much as a check on JAMA data as a data source in its own right. That is, I examined all the materials on chiropractic that were published in this journal in terms of format, style, content and themes, and compared this with the JAMA data. Had I found major differences -- such as a positive stance towards chiropractic or a surge of interest in chiropractic in the 1950s, when JAMA is silent -- I would have explored this and attempted to understand the difference. However, the BMSJ/NEJM data, such as it is, basically supported the JAMA data.

The BMSJ/NEJM data was located in a manner similar to the method used for JAMA. During the early years (up through 1930), when chiropractic was not always listed in the index, I examined the materials listed under the following index categories: Editorials, Miscellany, Legislation, Quackery, Correspondence and Spine.

Items regarding chiropractic that were published in the journal *Medical Economics* (ME) were analyzed through the years from 1955 to 1976. ME began in 1923 as a "throwaway" journal designed to cover issues of economic relevance to physicians such as practice building, financial planning and the use of allied health personnel. Unlike most medical publications, ME is not affiliated with any particular medical society or organization. I selected ME because of its position as an independent journal concerned with the economic interests of physicians. I anticipated that the items published in such a journal would offer the most open expressions of opposition to chiropractic. Articles were searched under the following index headings: Chiropractic, Allied Occupations, and Professionals, Other.

A final primary data source was the index of *AMA News* (AMAN), which changed to *American Medical News* (AMN) in 1969. AMAN/AMN is a newspaper published by the American Medical Association to cover many of the nonscientific items of interest for which there is only limited space in JAMA. The AMAN/AMN indices were searched under the heading "Chiropractic" from 1958 to 1976 and the titles of the articles so listed were analyzed by topic. Since AMAN/AMN is published by the AMA, I did not expect the thrust of its publications regarding chiropractic to differ substantially from those of JAMA. However, I wanted to examine this empirically and deemed an analysis of indexed titles regarding chiropractic to be sufficient for these purposes.

A variety of other primary data sources were used. For example, two books written by longtime JAMA editor Morris Fishbein, *Medical Follies* (1925) and *A History of the American Medical Association 1847 to 1947* (1947), provide additional data on the issues of general concern to the AMA and on the AMA's reaction to chiropractic in particular. A number of publications issued by the AMA for medical and public consumption, such as the pamphlets that were issued during the 1960s, were also examined.

Miscellaneous journal publications directed at physicians and other health workers were examined, such as materials published in *Student Physician, American Journal of Public Health,* and numerous other medical publications.

Secondary Data Sources

Many histories and analyses of U.S. medicine and the AMA were used to establish the social context within which the efforts of organized medicine to define chiropractic as deviant could be understood. The major references for the history and analysis of U.S. medicine include: Odin W. Anderson's *Health Services in the United States: A Growth Enterprise Since 1875* (1985); Joseph F. Kett's *The Formation of the American Medical Profession* (1968); Richard Harrison Shryock's *The Development of Modern Medicine* (1974); and Paul Starr's *The Social Transformation of American Medicine* (1982).

The major references for the history and analysis of the AMA (in addition to the primary data sources) include: James G. Burrow's *Organized Medicine in the Progressive Era* (1977) and *AMA: Voice of American Medicine* (1963); Oliver Garceau's *The Political Life of the American Medical Association* (1941); Hyde and Wolff's issue of the *Yale Law Journal* (1954); and Frank Campion's *The AMA and Health Policy Since 1940* (1984).

ISSUES REGARDING THE DATA

The data for this study consist of published communications regarding chiropractic by persons in the orthodox medical community. While a description of the data has been detailed above, there are several important issues that need to be addressed regarding the data and what it represents. These include the intention and function of the materials, the expressive and instrumental nature of the materials, the way information is conveyed through content, form and context, and the issue of whose viewpoint is expressed in these materials.

Intention and Function

The materials that I examined and analyzed have multiple intentions and serve multiple functions. Sometimes these intentions and functions overlap; sometimes they do not. I use the word "intention" to refer to the manifest or intended purpose of the material being published. The operative question here is: Why is this material being published? This question implies a particular point of view. Perhaps a more accurate formulation of the operative question is: According to the editors, why is this material being published? I use the word "function" to refer more to the possible consequences of the material presented. The operative question here is: What happens as a result of the material being published?[2]

I see three main intentions behind the publication of materials regarding chiropractic in medical journals: to provide information, to persuade or reconfirm a point of view, and to exhort to action. Any given piece may be published with one or all of these intentions. For example, in an editorial published in JAMA in August 1960, entitled "What Chiropractic Really Is Like! (In California, That Is)," all three intentions appear to be operating. The editorial begins:

> The cult of chiropractic does not, according to a recent report of the Stanford Research Institute, carry its weight as one of the methods of meeting the health needs of the community. Chiropractic is not a "great, uncrowded profession," as chiropractic publicists would have prospective students believe. Many of those in practice are doing so poorly that they have to supplement their income by other employment.[3]

Here the editorial clearly provides information to the reader: a summary of some "facts" about chiropractic in California. The next five paragraphs of the editorial present more information from the report. But the purpose of this item, as is true of all editorials, is to persuade and/or confirm a point of view. For any physicians who may feel sympathetic to chiropractors, this piece is designed to convince them otherwise and for physicians who are already opposed to chiropractic, this piece is designed to reconfirm that point of view. The last paragraph of this editorial reads:

> From time to time the *Journal* will publish some of the details from this most complete indictment of chiropractic as a claimed valid method of treating the sick. State medical societies having problems which involve chiropractic efforts to achieve state licensure and expanded recognition will be able to utilize the facts to show legislatures that this cult is not a worthwhile thing for the health and welfare of the people and that recognition of it certainly is not in their best interests.[4]

This part of the editorial provides a gentle but clear exhortation to action.

Imputing the intentions of actors can admittedly be a difficult business. In some cases, however, intentions seem fairly straightforward. Editorials, by definition, are written to present a point of view and convince others to adopt it by virtue of the argument presented. An item about the conviction of a chiropractor for practicing medicine without a license that is published in the "Medical News" section is on the face of it intended to relay a piece of information. When a letter to the editor is published that asks all physicians to write to legislators opposing a piece of chiropractic legislation, this is very clearly a call for action.

It is not always that easy to identify intentions and even when it is possible to identify *some* intentions, all intentions of a multiple-intentioned publication may not be identified. Furthermore, writers and editors themselves might not explicitly recognize their own intentions. How then can a sociologist analyzing these publications three-quarters of a century later hope to validly impute the intentions of this work? I have two answers to this question. First, I argue that this might be difficult if a particular item were seen and examined in isolation. But when a particular item is examined in the context in which it is published, intention may be more apparent. This can happen in analysis when one item becomes "an instance of" a phenomenon and the additional information one has about the phenomenon can then be brought to bear on the particular case. For example, when there are numerous reports of chiropractors being convicted, this fact provides more information -- and tells us something else about intentions -- than any single such report does alone.

Second, I argue that intention is not the only important point to be assessed regarding any given item. Switching attention from the authors and publishers to the audience or readers allows one to focus on function (as opposed to intention). The focus thus becomes the consequence of the material. The significance of material that is published lies in what this publication means to the publisher as audience (which is conceptually distinct from the publisher's intentions) and in what this means to the reader as audience. This latter point is similar to the distinction made by communications scholars who argue that the way in which a message is understood and used by the receiver should be studied (more than any preconceived effects).

This, of course, could present another analytical difficulty: How can a sociologist analyzing these publications three-quarters of a century later understand how these publications were interpreted and utilized by their audiences? Here I argue first that immersion in the primary data sources and information gleaned from the variety of secondary sources provides a basis for some degree of understanding of how these pieces are used and interpreted. But I also argue, in the functionalist tradition, that "the proof is in the pudding." That is, the use of these publications by the publishing audience (e.g. the leadership of the AMA) and the reading audience (e.g. the AMA member or subscriber) can be identified through the detailed study of the published materials, the social context of these publications and the relationship between the two. In other words, this can best be tapped by doing just the type of study I have done.

I do not view medical readers as passive vessels whose views regarding chiropractic are purely determined by the content of the medical articles they read on this subject. Certainly many physicians were influenced by the negative material published about chiropractic. It is also clear, however, that throughout this century some physicians were sympathetic to the idea of at least a limited place for chiropractic treatment in the panoply of healing therapies (see Gibbons 1981). The total acceptance of the content of the medical publications regarding chiropractic was not necessary for the publication of these materials to affect the social development of medicine. I argue that the perceived need for medical unity was one factor that was behind the intense opposition to chiropractic at various points in history; indeed, I argue that chiropractic was targeted *because* of the high degree of consensus regarding its undesirability. But the process of the deviantization of chiropractic went forward whether there were a few dissenters or not. Unity was not essential. It was the process of striving for unity that is important here.

Expressive and Instrumental Purposes

The publication of negative items regarding chiropractic serves both expressive and instrumental functions for orthodox medicine. Sometimes the materials published seem clearly expressive, as when an editorial rants against the "absurdity" of chiropractic. Other materials seem more clearly instrumental, as when an editorial calls for all physicians to tell their patients to vote against a chiropractic initiative. But while the expressive and instrumental functions of the publications are analytically distinct, they are integrally related in effect. The expressive aspect of these publications is the more relevant in my analysis, for it is through this expression that the issues of unity, status and dominance of orthodox medicine are forged and reaffirmed. But it is then this same unity, status and dominance that allow orthodox medicine to secure the concrete resources that come with high status and medical dominance (a very instrumental end).

Content and Form (or Text and Context)

The data are analyzed with respect to both content and form. As Richard

Brown notes (1983, p. 144), "Normally the denotative, explicit aspects of a text convey the informational content, whereas the commitment or relationship aspect is conveyed implicitly or even nonverbally by the manner or context of the text." The substance and manner of presentation of the materials published regarding chiropractic are analyzed at the beginning of chapters 3, 4 and 5.

The Data: Whose Viewpoint?

In any analysis of written documents, an important part of understanding what those documents represent is understanding the point of view that is expressed therein. This is particularly important in this study, because the major primary data sources and two other primary sources are official publications of medical professional associations (JAMA, NEJM, and AMN). Since JAMA is the major data source for this project, I will address this issue in some detail.

JAMA and the AMA JAMA has been the official publication of the AMA since the AMA switched to this weekly publication format in 1883. Although the AMA publishes many other medical journals, JAMA remains the primary publication and has the largest journal circulation. To understand the viewpoint that was represented in JAMA it is necessary to look at the extent to which JAMA reflected the positions of the AMA leadership, the extent to which the AMA leadership reflected the positions of the AMA membership, and the extent to which the AMA membership reflected the population of physicians practicing in the U.S.

I think it is clear that JAMA reflected the position of the AMA leadership. JAMA, as the official publication of the AMA, published materials that the leadership of the AMA chose to publish. The editor, in particular, exercised a great deal of influence over the content of JAMA (see the following section on Morris Fishbein). The Council and Section leaders were also influential as they decided on the content of their reports, which were then published in JAMA. I think, too, an argument can be made that once a position was published in JAMA it was seen as and treated as an official position of the AMA leadership (which is the more important issue as far as this particular study is concerned).

The issue of whether or not the AMA leadership truly represented the AMA membership is a more controversial topic. Social analysts have tended to doubt this representativeness while the AMA has tended to promote this representativeness.

Oliver Garceau (1941) analyzed the workings of the AMA across most of the first four decades of this century. He found no evidence of a long-tenured "active minority" ruling in the AMA House of Delegates, but he did find that the members of the AMA Councils, the trustees, the members of the standing committees and the AMA officers (except the president and vice president) tended to serve for very long periods of time. For example, between 1907 and 1938, the majority of members on the Council on Medical Education and Hospitals had between ten and twenty years or more tenure; the majority of members on the Council on Pharmacy and Chemistry had nineteen years or more tenure (Garceau 1941, p. 48). Additionally, Garceau found that many physicians served in several capacities at the same time or served in several offices consecutively.

There have been no major quantitative studies of the AMA since Garceau's work in 1941, but recent historical descriptive studies of the AMA provide some illustrations of these same leadership patterns, indicating that they continued across the decades of the 1950s, 1960s, and 1970s (although with unknown frequency). Campion (1984, chapter 8) calls this "moving through the chairs." For example, F.J.L. Blasingame, who was AMA Executive Vice President from 1958 to 1969, followed a long path of AMA involvement before reaching that top position. Starting with activity and leadership at the state level, he became an AMA delegate, a trustee, and Vice Chairman of the Board of Trustees before assuming the head staff position at the AMA (Campion 1984, p. 200). Likewise, James H. Sammons, who became Executive Vice President in 1974, had a similarly active career at the state level, became state delegate to the AMA in 1964, a trustee in 1970, a Vice Chairman of the Board, and was Chairman of the Board before assuming the executive vice presidency (Campion 1984, pp. 374-376). Sammons had won the executive vice presidency in a particularly unpleasant contest between himself and Richard S. Wilbur. Wilbur also illustrates the AMA leadership pattern. Wilbur had served as the deputy executive vice president, was grandson of the 1923 AMA President (who had also been chairman of the AMA Council on Medical Education for seventeen years) and was the nephew of the 1968 AMA president (who had himself been a delegate and trustee for many years) (Campion 1984, p. 371). The point here is that the incumbents of leadership positions in the AMA did in fact include many physicians who had been active in the organization for many years and who tended to keep their position for a long time. These leadership positions required a commitment and investment of time that an "average physician" might be unable to make. Campion (1984, p. 99) estimates that a member of the Board of Trustees currently spends at least 56 hours per year on association business. Considering that travel time would have added a significant amount of time to that figure earlier in this century, it is clear that this type of participation would systematically be out of the question for many types of physicians. These AMA leaders are thus not necessarily representative of the AMA membership at large.

Garceau (1941, pp. 51-53) found that those who were active in the AMA were not representative of all AMA members or all U.S. physicians: they were more likely to be urban, more likely to be specialists, and more likely to be academicians.

The leaders of the AMA itself tend to promote the idea that AMA policies really do express the wishes of the AMA membership. As I noted in chapter 2, the AMA was reorganized in 1901 to have state medical societies elect delegates to represent them in the AMA House of Delegates. While the AMA executives and the Board of Trustees have sometimes exerted much influence on AMA policy, the House of Delegates is technically the policy-making body of the AMA. This fact was very much part of the AMA rhetoric that the AMA was indeed the voice of American medicine. Garceau (1941, p. 28) noted this as he quoted from a Speaker's address to the House of Delegates in 1938:

> There can be no autocracy where final decision rests in a house composed of 175 delegates. There is no dictator among your officers. There is no dictator among the trustees to whom you delegate care of your money. There is no policy you may not reverse.... Thus the House of Delegates is convenient to point to to indicate the democratic representativeness of the AMA.[5]

This emphasis on the representativeness of the AMA continues in the second half of this century as well. For example, a 1968 JAMA article prepared by the AMA Law Division entitled "Lobbying, Legislation, and the American Medical Association" reiterates the representative basis of AMA policy:

> All AMA statements to the Congress on pending legislation or other matters, are based upon the policies established by its Board of Trustees and its physician-elected 242-man House of Delegates. Through its resolution, the House of Delegates reflects the continuing evolution of the practice of medicine and medical thought.... The 215,000 physician-members of the AMA hold opinions that cover the entire spectrum of thought on any legislative proposal or question of policy. It is through the House of Delegates that these diverse opinions are combined into the single voice of AMA policy.[6]

While this quote mentions initial diversity among members of the AMA (which earlier essays did not acknowledge[7]), it reaffirms their view that policies of the AMA are constructed in a representative and democratic process.

The extent to which the AMA represents the population of physicians in the U.S. is also unclear. As I noted before, earlier in the century Garceau (1941, p. 48) found that those who were active in the AMA were more likely to be specialists and more likely to be academics than other AMA members or the general population of U.S. physicians. But Campion (1984, p. 52) notes that after World War I many academic physicians left the AMA over the state medicine issue (and stayed away) and that private practitioners came to dominate the association. Campion's recent comparison of AMA members with nonmembers also indicates office-based physicians are disproportionately represented in the AMA today (1984, p.54).

The proportion of U.S. physicians belonging to the AMA is also relevant here. In 1910, 50% of U.S. physicians belonged to the AMA. This increased to 60% in 1920, 65.1% in 1930, and, after a decline in 1935 to 60.8%, was up to 66.8% in 1940 (Burrow 1963, pp. 49-51; Garceau 1941, pp. 130-132). In 1982, after the difficult 1960s and 1970s, the membership rate was 45% (Campion 1984, p. 46), which is about where it is today as well.

In regard to how AMA membership relates to the reading of AMA publications, it appears that nonmembers are still quite likely to read AMA publications. A JAMA readership survey done in 1950[8] found that JAMA was read by two times as many physicians as any other medical journal. The survey found that 77% of all practicing physicians read JAMA on a "regular basis" and that this did not vary by AMA membership (or by age, type of practice, specialty or residence). AMAN circulation was reported to be 269,568 as of June 30, 1960, which was "more than any other medical publication aimed at physicians."[9] A 1960 AMAN readership survey found that 90% of U.S. physicians read it "regularly," which means that physicians who were not AMA members were nonetheless reading AMAN.[10]

For my purposes, the most important issues are not whether or not the AMA leadership "really" expresses the views of its members or whether the AMA membership "really" is representative of U.S. physicians or the profession of medicine as a whole in the U.S. This analysis focuses on the internal organizational activities of the AMA (and to a lesser extent other elements of organized medicine) and the relation of these activities to the profession of medicine as it attempted to secure that title ("profession") and all that it means in terms of status and dominance. What the AMA published is part of that process. Therefore, I look at the issue of the representativeness of the AMA in terms of how the AMA officially promoted the view that its policies did in fact reflect the voice and interest of its members and American medicine in general (and ultimately the interests of the public's health). I see the issue of representativeness as being integrally linked to the promotion of unity by the AMA, the unity that is seen as so central to the establishment and maintenance of occupational status and dominance of medicine (and of which the deviantization of chiropractic is so centrally a part).

Morris Fishbein: Moral Entrepreneur? It is important to consider the possibility that publication of anti-chiropractic material in JAMA was really only a reflection of the particular and personal interests of the JAMA editor or other leaders in the AMA; that is, that opposition to chiropractic in the pages of JAMA was merely a reflection of the particular interests of a particular entrepreneur. I will address this suggestion and show why it is an inadequate explanation.

Becker (1963) coined the term moral entrepreneur in his efforts to explain the creation of marijuana use as a deviant category. He defines the term moral entrepreneur in terms of rule creation:

> Rules are the products of someone's initiative and we can think of the people who exhibit such enterprise as moral entrepreneurs. (emphasis omitted)

But we can easily and usefully extend the concept to include those who promote certain definitions that then allow for new rules to be created.

Becker argues that Harry Anslinger, Commissioner of Narcotics, was such an entrepreneur in his efforts to outlaw marijuana. Although others, such as Dickson (1968), have argued that Becker missed the organizational basis behind the movement to outlaw marijuana, the concept of moral entrepreneur has remained a useful tool for sociologists interested in explaining the creation of deviance. Bustamante (1972) applied and expanded the concept of moral entrepreneur to the deviantization of illegal Mexican laborers in the U.S. Ben-Yehuda (1985) used the concept to characterize the role of the authors of the *Malleus Maleficarum* in the European witchcraze in the late 1400s.

There have been several individuals involved in the social construction of chiropractic as deviant that can perhaps be classified as moral entrepreneurs. First and foremost is the late Morris Fishbein. Fishbein became assistant editor of JAMA in 1913 and served as JAMA editor from 1924 to 1949. The personal influence of Morris Fishbein cannot be overstated. Journalist Milton Mayer (1949, pp. 76-77) noted the references to Fishbein as "Dr. AMA" and the AMA as the "American Fishbein Association." Twenty-five years later historian Frank Campion (1984, p. 114) echoed this, writing that "for over two decades, Fishbein *was* the AMA" (emphasis in the original).

Fishbein was responsible for many of the early vituperative diatribes against chiropractic. Odin Anderson (1985, p. 101, n. 14) kindly referred to Fishbein's writing as "colorful," saying that Fishbein "loved words and was a good phrase maker." Others, not so kind, referred to his "low-comedy routine" (Mayer 1949). And quackery was clearly one of Fishbein's favorite topics; he wrote the book *Medical Follies* in 1925.

It may be tempting to suggest that all the fuss about chiropractic by the AMA in the pages of JAMA was really only the result of the moral entrepreneurship of a powerful voice in the AMA. But such an argument cannot be supported. Morris Fishbein retired as editor of JAMA in 1949, but the intense opposition to chiropractic in the pages of JAMA had ended seven years before (and had stopped long before that, except for the brief "spurt" again from 1936 to 1942). When the intensity increased again in the 1960s and 1970s, Fishbein had been long gone. Blasingame, who was executive vice president of the AMA throughout the 1960s, and Sabatier, head of the Committee on Quackery, could perhaps also be considered moral entrepreneurs. But when we begin to see such strings of moral entrepreneurship or variations in moral entrepreneurship, we must look (as Dickson did) for the social sources of such activities. That is exactly what I have attempted to do in this book.

Even without the inspiring spirit of moral entrepreneurship, the possibility of the systematic bias of editors must be considered. There were eight JAMA editors between 1908 and 1976, the period under scrutiny in this book. The first two editors both had very long tenures. George H. Simmons was the editor for 25 years, from February 1899 to September 1924, and Morris Fishbein followed him for the next 25 years, from September 1924 to December 1949. Austin Smith served as editor from December 1949 to December 1958, followed by a brief tenure by Johnson F. Hammond, who served less than a year from December 1958 to October 1959. John H. Talbott was editor from October 1959 to 1969. He was followed by Hugh Hussey, serving from 1969 to October 1973, Robert H. Moser, October 1973 to June 1975, and William R. Barclay, who began his tenure in June 1975 and served for the remaining year and a half under consideration here.[11] These dates of editorial tenure do not correspond to the three stages of medical response to chiropractic that I outline in the previous chapters (1908 to 1924, 1925 to 1960, and 1961 to 1976). Nor do they correspond to the sheer quantity of medical materials published regarding chiropractic across this century. Particular editors do have their biases, but these do not appear to account for the historical variations in the response to chiropractic.

ISSUES REGARDING THE METHODOLOGY

My study is basically a social historical study using the logic and methods of qualitative sociological research. I looked at how the construction of a particular social world was related to the social structures within which it was being constructed and lived.

Diesing (1971, p. 7) notes that the methods used by some historians "to reconstruct a whole historical period out of available data and try to understand it, intuitively or 'from the inside,' as a kind of integrated system" is really a type of participant-observer method. But he warns that an historical period does not constitute "a self-maintaining system with actual boundaries; even if it were, it would be much too large to reconstruct in all its inner workings" (1971, p.7). This is an important point. Although I have read primary and secondary sources extensively to better grasp the social worlds of physicians in general and physicians in organized medicine in particular, my grasp of these worlds is necessarily circumscribed by the limits of the data sources and the enormity of the task.

I use the term "qualitative" to describe my research methods for two main reasons. First, I was basically engaged in theory-generating rather than theory-testing. I approached my subject matter first and my analysis is grounded in this data (Glaser and Strauss 1967). Second, I approached my data holistically, which basically means I assumed that each element could only be understood in the context of the whole (Diesing 1971). Although I have very simply quantified some of my data, I have used that information in the qualitative tradition of considering it one more piece of information that is part of the whole.

Procedures

Like any theory-generating qualitative study, mine was a study involving ongoing discovery and verification in the course of systematically examining and re-examining data. Diesing (1971, p. 15) notes that in this type of study "*[j]ustification and verification* are not treated as a separate set of procedures *after* 'discovery,' but are included *within* the process of discovery" (emphasis in the original). To verify or discount working hypotheses, I typically went back to the same data sets to reexamine or recode with the new questions in mind.

For my purposes, I generally viewed the materials published in the editorial sections of the journals and in full or special articles as being the most significant. In part, this was an *a priori* decision on my part, since editorial sections are designed to present the official point of view and full articles are published only on topics that are seen as significant by the editors. These are the sections where the rhetoric and accounts that constitute the deviantization of chiropractic are seen most clearly.

These two sections are also among the most widely read sections in JAMA. A 1950 readership survey, for example, found that the six most widely read sections of JAMA were (in rank order): Table of Contents, Original Articles, Editorials and Comments, Current Medical Literature, Clinical Notes, and Queries and Minor Notes.[12] Both the Editorials and Comments sections and, frequently, the Queries and Minor Notes sections include editorial commentary.

The first steps in my project involved identifying general themes that came up in the data. Next I looked more closely at how these themes were handled, the context in which the theme is raised, and so forth, always looking for variations and using these variations as signals of issues that needed to be pursued. Some of these themes were substantive text themes and some of these were presentational or context themes. On the basis of this analysis I initially recognized the three distinct stages in the response of organized medicine to chiropractic. This was then modified based on a division that allowed me to best make sense of the data.[13]

The next step in my data analysis was to look at how the medical responses to chiropractic that I had identified could be linked to the other elements of the historical context within which organized medicine was operating (and physicians were living). Here I used information in my primary and secondary data sources to identify possible relevant events and interpretations of events that might in part account for the differential response to chiropractic across the twentieth century. This again was a matter of continual discovery and verification, as I looked for factors that could account for increases when there were increases, decreases when there were decreases, and ruled out a variety of plausible alternative hypotheses.

CONCLUSION

In his book *Historical Sociology* (1982, p. 108) the late Philip Abram notes that the tendency for social scientists to move beyond their data and methods is very strong:

> The temptation to move from the discovery (or construction) of pattern and probability within given historical configurations of action and structure to the assertion of supra-historical causal sequence or destiny is very strong.

The task of the historical sociologist, however, is to discern the specifically *historical structuring* of action without falling into the trap of separating structure from action or postulating a theory of history in which a succession of structural types - like the parade of ghostly kings in Macbeth - has an existence independent of the creation of structure through action. (emphasis in the original)

Following Abram, I have worked hard to fully plumb the richness of my data for what it can contribute to our understanding of the social world that is constructed by physicians in their collective association in the AMA. I have tried to go one step further and explore how this social world is part of the broader social structural setting in which it exists and of which it is a part. My data and methods allow me to go no further.

NOTES

1.   Five chiropractors in Illinois, home of the AMA, filed an anti-trust suit against fifteen medical associations and four physicians in the AMA (including two chairs of the AMA's Committee on Quackery). The national medical associations named in the suit were: the AMA, the American hospital Association, the American College of Surgeons, the American College of Physicians, the Joint Commission on the Accreditation of Hospitals, the American College of Radiology, the American Academy of Orthopedic Surgeons, the American Osteopathic Association and the American Academy of Physical Medicine and Rehabilitation. The suit also named several medical associations in Illinois: the Illinois State Medical Society, the Chicago Medical Society, and the Medical Society of Cook County. See Wardwell (1982) for a summary of the initial filing of *Wilk, C.A. et al. v AMA et al.* (Complaint #76C3777, Oct. 12, 1976, US District Court, Northern District of Illinois, Eastern Division) and Wardwell (1992) for a discussion of the case conclusion. Although the court found the defendants not guilty in 1981, this decision was appealed and was overturned by a US District Court ruling in 1987. By then the chiropractors had already reached out-of-court settlements with several of the defendant associations and the AMA had already changed its Code of Ethics to allow professional relations between physicians and chiropractors. The AMA lost its appeal of the 1987 ruling in 1990.

2.   I am thus using these terms somewhat differently from Merton (1949), who spoke of both intention and function is relation to consequences. In some ways I am doing both "manifest content analysis" (Berelson 1952), which is basically looking what there is without making references, and "propaganda analysis" (George 1959), which is looking at what is between the lines and making inferences.

3.   JAMA Aug. 6, 1960, 173(14):1582.

4.   JAMA Aug.6, 1960, 173(14):1582.

5. JAMA July 2, 1938, p. 32, as quoted in Garceau (1941, p. 28).

6. JAMA Sept. 23, 1968, 205(13):218. Prepared by the AMA Law Division (by Charles W. Pahl).

7. Garceau (1941) and Hyde and Wolff (1954) and even Fishbein (1947) himself point to the efforts of the AMA to put forth a front of unity and unanimity.

8. JAMA Dec. 21, 1950, 144(8):633.

9. JAMA Oct. 22, 1960, 174(8):1042.

10. *Ibid.*

11. Sources for the editorship information are: JAMA July 28, 1969, 209(4):487; JAMA Nov. 8, 1976, 236(19):2212; and Campion (1984, pp. 490-497).

12. JAMA Dec. 21, 1950, 144(8):663.

13. The decision to divide the response of organized medicine to chiropractic into three periods was thus based on the data only (not on any other information regarding orthodox medicine in general or organized medicine in particular). The particular beginning and end points for each period were identified based on a subjective decision regarding how well the materials published about chiropractic "fit together" within each period. This decision was based on the content of the publications, the number and types of items published, and the manner of presentation of the material.

Appendix B

Medical Publications: Supporting Data

This appendix is comprised of the variety of systematically collected data which supports the analyses and conclusions in this book. The tables and figures below are those to which reference is made throughout the book.

Figure 1

Number of Chiropractic Items Published in JAMA Per Year

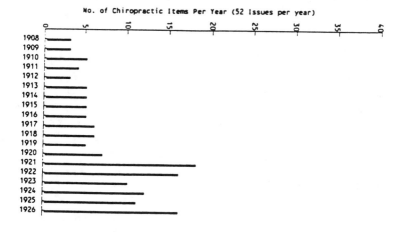

No. of Chiropractic Items Per Year (52 issues per year)

Figure 1 Continued

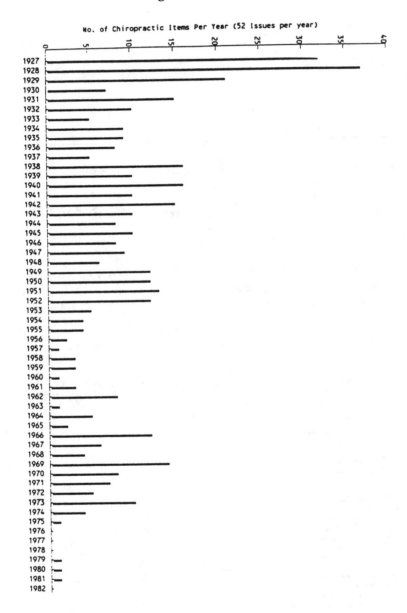

Table 1

Type of Chiropractic Items Published in JAMA Per Year

	TOTAL	Article/Social Report	Editorial	Current Comment	Medicolegal/Law & Medicine	Correspondence/Q & A/Letters / Queries & Minor Notes	Medical News/Wash. News/ AMAgrams	Miscellaneous *
1908	3						1	2
1909	3						2	1
1910	5						3	2
1911	4				4			
1912	3				1			2
1913	5			1	3	1		
1914	5			1	4			
1915	5	1			3			1
1916	5			1	4			
1917	6			1	1			4
1918	6			1	3			2
1919	5			1	3			1
1920	7			4	1		1	1
1921	18	1		6	2	6	1	2
1922	16		1	6	5	1	1	2
1923	10		1	1	1		1	6
1924	12			6	2	3		1
1925	11	1	1	1	6		1	1
1926	16			3	4	1	7	1
1927	32			3	5		22	2
1928	37						33	4
1929	21	1	1		2		15	2
1930	7				1		4	2
1931	15			1	7		5	2
1932	10		1	1	3		4	1
1933	5				3		1	1
1934	9		1		3		3	2
1935	9				5		3	1

Table 1 Continued

	TOTAL	Article/Social Report	Editorial	Current Comment	Medicolegal/Law & Medicine	Correspondence/Q & A/Letters	Queries & Minor Notes/	Medical News/Wash. News/ AMAgrams	Miscellaneous *
1936	8				5			2	1
1937	5				2			1	2
1938	16		3		6	1		2	4
1939	10				6	1		1	2
1940	16		1	1	8	1			5
1941	10		1		4				5
1942	15		2	1	4			4	4
1943	10				6			2	2
1944	8			1	4			1	2
1945	10				3			4	3
1946	8				2			2	4
1947	9	1		1	3			1	3
1948	6				2			1	3
1949	12			1	3	1		1	6
1950	12				8			1	3
1951	13				4	1		2	6
1952	12				8				4
1953	5				3				2
1954	4				1			1	2
1955	4				2				2
1956	2				1				1
1957	1				1				
1958	3				1				2
1959	3	1					1		1
1960	1		1						
1961	3						1	1	1
1962	8							6	2
1963	1								1
1964	5	1	1				1	1	1
1965	2							2	

Table 1 Continued

	TOTAL	Article/Social Report	Editorial	Current Comment	Medicolegal/Law & Medicine	Correspondence/Q & A/Letters	Queries & Minor Notes/AMAgrams	Medical News/Wash. News/AMAgrams	Miscellaneous*
1966	12	1				1	1	8	1
1967	6	1					1	2	2
1968	4					1		3	
1969	14		2			3		9	
1970	8		1			1	3	2	1
1971	7	1	1				1	4	
1972	5		2				1	2	
1973	10		1			2		7	
1974	4	1						3	
1975	1							1	
1976	1							1	
1977	0								
1978	0								
1979	1								1
1980	1	1							
1981	1							1	
1982	0								

* - Medical Economics
- Propoganda for Reform
- Medical Education and State
    Boards of Registration
- Association News
- Foreign Letters
- Officers' Reports
- Medical Licensure Statistics
- AMA Organization Section
- Medical Education, Registration
    and Hospital Service
- Annual Reports of Board of Trustees

Table 2

Titles from Medicolegal Section of JAMA*
First Chiropractic-Related Title Appearing Each Year, 1925-1960,
State Noted

1925	Chiropractic College Liable for Injuries by Students (OK)
1926	Chiropractic and the Illinois Medical Practice Act (IL)
1927	Action Against Intruder into Profession - "Treatment" (AL)
1928	- None -
1929	Regulation of Conferring of Degrees (NJ)
1930	Electric Treatments by Chiropractor Unlawful (NJ)
1931	Evidence: Chiropractor as an Expert Witness (Federal)
1932	Insurance, Health: Chiropractor Not a "Licensed Physician or Surgeon" (MI)
1933	Malpractice: Right of Physician to Testify Against Chiropractor Using Diathermy Medicine (CA)
1934	Medical Practice Acts: Electrical Treatments Administered by a Chiropractor (NJ)
1935	Insurance, Life: Chiropractor Not a "Physician" (MI)
1936	Malpractice: Acute Urethritis Following Instrumentation by a Drugless Practitioner (CA)
1937	Malpractice; Death Resulting from Chiropractic Treatment for Headache (FL)
1938	Chiropractic: Death of Patient from Cerebral hemorrhage Following Treatment (MA)
1939	Medical Practice Acts: Injunction to Restrain Unlawful Practice (NY)
1940	Medical Practice Acts: Scope of Chiropractic in Iowa (IA)
1941	Medical Practice Acts: Right of Unlicensed Chiropractor to Question Constitutionality of Act (VA)
1942	Chiropractors: License a Prerequisite to Collection of Fees (TX)
1943	Chiropractors: Advertising as Evidence of Unlicensed Practice (OH)
1944	Medical Practice Acts: Unlicensed Practice of Medicine by Chiropractor (NJ)
1945	Malpractice: Explosion of Bulb in Infra-Red lamp (CA)
1946	Malpractice: Negligent Roentgen Examination by Chiropractor (CA)
1947	Chiropractor Practice Act: Board's Right to Cancel License Without Notice or Hearing, Reversal of Previous Decision (CA)

Table 2 (Continued)

Titles from Medicolegal Section of JAMA*
First Chiropractic-Related Title Appearing Each Year, 1925-1960,
State Noted

1948	Chiropractic Practice Acts: Validity of Annual Registration Prerequisite (WI)
1949	Chiropractic Practice Acts: Board May Not Waive Basic Science Act Requirements (AR)
1950	Chiropractic Practice Acts: length of College Course Required (GA)
1951	Building Restrictions: Right of Chiropractor to Maintain Office in Home (MD)
1952	Medical Practice Acts: Constitutionality of in Relation to Chiropractors (IN)
1953	Medical Practice Acts: Constitutionality as Applied to Chiropractors (LA)
1954	Workmen's Compensation Acts: Employee's Suit for Malpractice by Physician (CA)
1955	Roentgenograms: Performance of X-ray Services for Chiropractors (NY)
1956	Building Restrictions: Right of Chiropractic to Maintain Office in Home (MD)
1957	Chiropractors: Injunction to Prevent Unlicensed Practice (IL)
1958	Use of Oscilloclast as Fraud in Practice of Medicine (CA)
1959	- None -
1960	- "Medicolegal Abstracts" no longer published in JAMA -

*Sources: Titles are from the following issues of JAMA:

Apr. 18, 1925, 84(16):1235-6.
Jan. 30, 1926, 86(5):371.
Mar. 19, 1927, 88(12):953.
May 11, 1929, 92(19):1627.
Sept. 13, 1930, 95(11):822.
Mar. 7, 1931, 96(10):802.
Jan. 16, 192, 98(3):256.
Mar. 11, 1933, 100(10):770.
Apr. 7, 1934, 102(14): 1185.
Feb. 16, 1935, 104(7);590.

Jan. 25, 1936, 106(4):323.
July 17, 1937, 109(3):233.
July 26, 1938, 110(9):683-4.
Feb. 11, 1939, 112(6):576.
Mar. 2, 1940, 114(9):826.
May 3, 1941, 116(18):2103.
Jan. 10, 1942, 118(2):166.
Jan. 9, 1943, 121(2):150.
Apr. 29, 1944, 124(18):1315.
Feb. 10, 1945, 127(6):355.

Apr. 27, 1946, 130(17):1262-3.
Mar. 1, 1947, 133(9):646.
June 26, 1948, 137(9):810.
Jan. 15, 1949, 139(3):177.
Apr. 8, 1950, 142(14):1099.
June 30, 1951, 146(9):866-7.
Jan. 12, 1952, 148(2):137.
Jan. 3, 1953, 151(1):66-7.

Aug. 28, 1954, 155(18):1602.
June 25, 1955, 158(8):693.
June 30, 1956, 161(9):902.
June 22, 1957, 164(8):918.
May 3, 1958, 167(1):101-2.

Figure 2

**Number of Chiropractic Items in JAMA Each Year with Editorial Content
(Includes Articles/Special Reports, Editorials, Current Comment, and Queries and Minor Notes)**

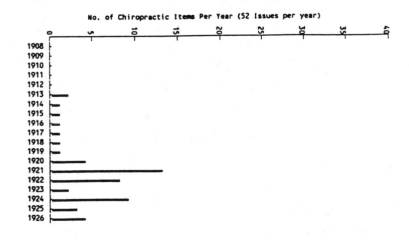

Figure 2 Continued

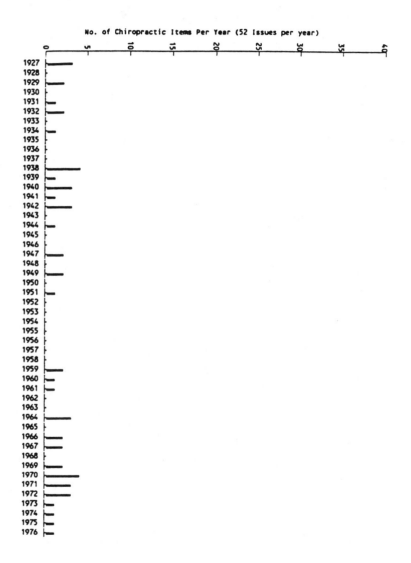

No. of Chiropractic Items Per Year (52 Issues per year)

Figure 3

Number of Chiropractic Items in BMSJ/NEJM Per Year

No. of Chiropractic Items per Year (52 issues per year)

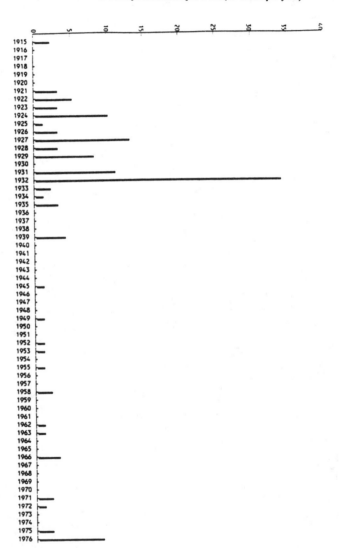

Table 2

Type of Chiropractic Items Published in BMSJ/NEJM Per Year

Year	Total	Original Article	Editorial	News item	"Miscellany" Editorial	Correspondence	Legislative	Other
1915	2		1		1			
1916	0							
1917	0							
1918	0							
1919	0							
1920	0							
1921	3		1		1			1
1922	5		1		2		1	1
1923	3		1		1	1		
1924	10		4	2	2	1	1	
1925	1							1
1926	3		1		1		1	
1927	13	1	3		3	2	4	
1928	3		1		2			
1929	8		4		2		2	
1930	0							
1931	11		5	1	1		4	
1932	34	1	8		6	14	4	1
1933	2				1		1	
1934	1						1	
1935	3							
1936	0							

Year	Total	Orig- inal Article	Edi- torial	News Item	"Miscel- lany" Editorial	Corre- spon- dance	Leg- isla- tive	Oth- er
1937	0							
1938	0							
1939	4		1				3	
1940	0							
1941	0							
1942	0							
1943	0							
1944	0							
1945	1							1
1946	0							
1947	0							
1948	0							
1949	1							
1950	0							
1951	0							
1952	1		1					
1953	1					1		
1954	0							
1955	1		1					
1956	0							
1957	0							
1958	2		2					
1959	0							
1960	0							

Year	Total	Orig-inal Article	Edi-torial	News Item	"Miscel-lany" Editorial	Corre-spon-dence	Leg-isla-tive	Oth-er
1961	0							
1962	1		1					
1963	1							
1964	0							
1965	0							
1966	3		2			1		
1967	0							
1968	0							
1969	0							
1970	0							
1971	2					2		
1972	1	1						
1973	0							
1974	0							
1975	2	1	1					
1976	9					9		

Table 3

Type of Chiropractic Items in *Medical Economics* Per Year

Year	Total	Original Article	Editorial	"News Item"	"Your World"	"Your Profession"
1955	3	1		2		
1956	3			3		
1957	2			2		
1958	1			1		
1959	4	1		3		
1960	2			2		
1961	2	2			*	*
1962	3	1			2	*
1963	1	1			*	
1964	2	2				*
1965	0					
1966	1	1				
1967	0					
1968	3	3				
1969	0					
1970	1	1				
1971	1	1				
1972	0					
1973	1	1				
1974	1					
1975	0					
1976	1	1				

* The item is article length and is included in the "Article" column.

Figure 4

Number of Chiropractic Items in *AMA News/American Medical News* Per Year

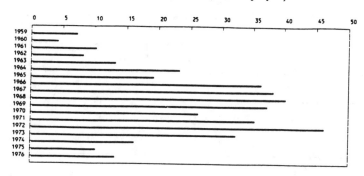

No. of Chiropractic Items per Year (52 issues per year)

Table 4

Number of Items Indexed Under Heading "Chiropractic" in *AMA News/American Medical News* **Per Year**

Year	Number of Items
1959	7
1960	4
1961	10
1962	8
1963	13
1964	23
1965	19
1966	36
1967	38
1968	40
1969	37
1970	26
1971	32
1972	44
1973	31
1974	16
1975	10
1976	13

Table 5

Type of Chiropractic Items in *AMA News/American Medical News* Per Year

Year	Regulation of Chiropractic	Cases of Chiropractors	Reports of Wrongdoing by Chiropractors Causing Injury	Insurance Coverage of Chiropractic	Chiropractic Coverage under Federal Program	Chiropractic Suits Against AMA and Others	General Negative Against Chiropractic	Other
1959	7							
1960	2							2
1961	6							3
1962	5	1	1		1			
1963	4	1	3		2			3
1964	9	2	7	1	2	2		
1965	9	1	3		2		1	3
1966	10	2	6		2	1	2	13
1967	6	2	5	1	15		6	3
1968	10	4	8	1	5	2	5	5
1969	7		6	4	8	2	6	4
1970	3		1	1	13	1	4	3
1971	2		2	5	7		5	11
1972	4			5	9	1	7	18
1973	3		3		7	1	2	15
1974	3				5			8
1975	3		1			1		4
1976	5		2			1		5

References

Abrams, Philip. 1982. *Historical Sociology*. Ithaca, NY: Cornell University Press.

Albrecht, Gary L. and Judith A. Levy. 1982. "The Professionalization of Osteopathy: Adaptation in the Medical Marketplace." Pp. 161-206 in *Research in the Sociology of Health Care*, vol. 2, edited by J. A. Roth. Greenwich, CT: JAI Press.

AMA. 1993. *Medical Groups: A Comparative Analysis*. Chicago, IL: American Medical Association, as reported in Mike Mitka, "AMA Study Says Group Practices Pay Moore, but Make Patients Wait," *American Medical News*, March 7, 1994, 37(9):4.

Anderson, Odin W. 1985. *Health Services in the United States: A Growth Enterprise Since 1875*. Ann Arbor, MI: Health Administration Press.

Anderson, Robert T. 1981. "Medicine, Chiropractic and Caste." *Anthropological Quarterly* 54(3):157-165.

Ayers, Steven M. 1996. *Health Care in the United States: The Facts and the Choices*. Chicago: American Library Association.

Becker, Howard. 1963. Outsiders: *Studies in the Sociology of Deviance*. New York: Free Press.

------. 1962. "The Nature of Professions." Pp. 27-46 in *Education for the Professions*. Chicago: University of Chicago Press.

Begun, James W. and Ronald C. Lippincott. 1980. "The Politics of Professional Control: The Case of Optometry." Pp. 53-103 in *Research in the Sociology of Health Care*, vol. 1, edited by J. A. Roth. Greenwich, CT: JAI Press.

Ben-Yehuda, Nachman. 1985. *Deviance and Moral Boundaries: Witchcraft, the Occult, Science Fiction, Deviant Sciences and Scientists.* Chicago: University of Chicago Press.

Berelson, B. 1952. *Content Analysis in Communications Research.* New York: Free Press.

Berger, Peter L. and Thomas Luckmann. 1966. *The Social Construction of Reality.* Garden City, NJ: Doubleday/Anchor Books.

Berlant, Jeffrey Lionel. 1975. *Profession and Monopoly: A Study of Medicine in the United States and Great Britain.* Berkeley, CA: University of California Press.

Berman, Alex. 1978. "The Heroic Approach in 19th Century Therapeutics." Pp 77-86 in *Sickness and Health in America*, edited by J.W. Leavitt and R.L. Numbers. Madison, WI: University of Wisconsin Press.

Boston Women's Health Collective. 1973. *Our Bodies, Ourselves.* New York: Simon and Schuster.

Brown, E. Richard. 1979. *Rockefellar Medicine Men: Medicine and Capitalism in America.* Berkeley, CA: University of California Press.

Brown, Richard Harvey. 1983. "Theories of Rhetoric and the Rhetoric of Theories." *Social Research* 50(1): 126-157.

Burnham, John C. 1982. "American Medicine's Golden Age: What Happened to It?" *Science* 215 (March 19):1474-1479.

Burrow, James G. 1977. *Organized Medicine in the Progressive Era: The Move Toward Monopoly.* Baltimore: Johns Hopkins University Press.

------. 1963. *AMA: Voice of American Medicine.* Baltimore: Johns Hopkins University Press.

Bustamante, Jorge A. 1972. "The 'Wetback' as Deviant: An Application of Labeling Theory." *American Journal of Sociology* 77:706-718.

Campion, Frank D. 1984. *The AMA and U.S. Health Policy Since 1940.* Chicago: Chicago Review Press.

Chambliss, William. 1976. "Functional and Conflict Theories of Crime: The Heritage of Emile Durkheim and Karl Marx." Pp. 1-28 in *Whose Law? What Order?*, edited by W. J. Chambliss and M. Mankoff. New York: John Wiley & Sons.

Cobb, Ann Kuckelman. 1977. "Pluralistic Legitimation of an Alternative Therapy System: The Case of Chiropractic." *Medical Anthropolgy* 1(4):1-23.

Coburn, David and C. Lesley Biggs. 1986. "Limits to Medical Dominance: The Case of Chiropractic." *Social Science and Medicine* 22(10):1035-1046.

Deising, Paul. 1971. *Patterns of Discovery in the Social Sciences.* Chicago: Aldine-Atherton.

Deutsch, Ronald M. 1977. *The New Nuts Among the Berries.* Palo Alto, CA: Bull Publishing Co.

Dickson, Donald T. 1968. "Bureaucracy and Morality: An Organizational Perspective on a Moral Crusade." *Social Problems* 16:143-156.

Durkheim, Emile. [1895] 1962. *The Rules of Sociological Method.* 8th ed. Translated by S.A. Solovay and J.H. Mueller; edited by G.E.G. Catlin. Reprint, Glencoe, IL: Free Press.

------. [1893]1947. The Division of Labor in Society. Translated by G. Simpson. Reprint, Glencoe, IL: Free Press.

Dye, A. Augustus. [1939]1969. *The Evolution of Chiropractic.* Reprint, Richmond Hall (no location given).

Earle, A. Scott. 1969. "The Germ Theory in America: Antisepsis and Asepsis." *Surgery* 65:508-522.

Ehrenreich, Barbara and Diedre English. 1978. *For Her Own Good.* New York: Anchor/Doubleday.

Eisenberg, David M. and Roanld Kessler, Cindy Foster, Frances Norlock, David Calkins and Thomas Delbanco. 1993. "Unconventional Medicine in the United States: Prevalence, Costs, and Patterns of Use." *The New England Journal of Medicine* 328(4):246-252.

Erikson, Kai T. 1966. *Wayward Puritans.* New York: John Wiley & Sons.

Feldstein, Paul. 1977. *Health Associations and the Demand for Legislation: The Political Economy of Health.* Cambridge, MA: Ballinger.

Fishbein, Morris. 1947. *A History of the American Medical Association 1847-1947.* Philadelphia: W.B. Saunders Co.

------. 1925. *The Medical Follies.* New York: Boni and Liveright.

Fielding, Stephen L. 1984. "Organizational Impact on Medicine: The HMO Concept." *Social Science and Medicine* 18(8):615-620.

Freidson, Eliot. 1986. *Professional Powers: A Study of the Institutionalization of Formal Knowledge.* Chicago: University of Chicago Press.

------. 1971. *Profession of Medicine: A Study of the Sociology of Applied Knowledge.* New York: Dodd, Mead & Co.

------. 1970. *Professional Dominance: The Social Structure of Medical Care.* New York: Atherton.

Garceau, Oliver. 1941. *The Political Life of the American Medical Association.* Cambridge, MA: Harvard University Press.

George, Alexander L. 1959. *Propaganda Analysis: A Study of Inferences Made from Nazi Propaganda in World War II.* Evanston, IL: Row,

Peterson.

Gibbons, Russell W. 1993. "Minnesota, 1905: Who Killed the First Chiropractic Legislation?" *Chiropractic History* 13(1):27-32.

------. 1981. "Physician-Chiropractors: Medical Presence in the Evolution of Chiopractic." *Bulletin of the History of Medicine* 55:233-245.

------. 1980. "The Evolution of Chiropractic: Medical and Social Protest in America." Pp. 3-24 in *Modern Developments in the Principles and Practice of Chiropractic*, edited by S. Haldeman. New York: Appleton-Century-Crofts.

------. 1977. "Chiropractic History: Turbulence and Triumph: The Survival of A Profession." Pp. 139-148 in *Who's Who in Chiropractic, International 1976-1078*, edited by F.L. Dzaman. Littleton, CO: International Publishing Co.

Gilb, Corinne Lathrop. 1966. *Hidden Hierarchies*. New York: Harper and Row.

Gusfield, Joseph. 1963. *Symbolic Crusade: Status Politics and the American Temperance Movement*. Urbana, IL: University of Illinois Press.

Hall, Oswald. 1946. "The Informal Organization of the Medical Profession." *Canadian Journal of Economics and Political Science* 12(1):30-44.

Haug, Marie and Bebe Lavin. 1983. *Consumerism in Medicine*. Beverly Hills, CA: Sage Publications.

Haug, Marie and Marvin Sussman. 1969. "Professional Autonomy and the Revolt of the Client." *Social Problems* 17:153-161.

Hughes, Everett C. 1965. "Professions." Pp 1-14 in *The Professions in America*, edited by K.S. Lynn. Boston: Houghton Mifflin.

------. 1958. *Men and Their Work*. Glencoe, IL: Free Press.

Hyde, David R. and Payson Wolff, eds. 1954. "The American Medical Association: Power, Purpose, Politics in Organized Medicine." *Yale Law Journal* 68:938-1022.

Inverarity, James. 1980. "Theories of the Political Creation of Deviance: Legacies of Conflict Theory, Marx and Durkheim." Pp. 175-217 in *A Political Analysis of Deviance*, edited by P. Lauderdale. Minneapolis, MN: University of Minnesota Press.

------. 1976. "Population and Lynching in Louisiana, 1889-1896: A Test of Erikson's Theory of the Relationship Between Boundary Crises and Repressive Justice." *American Sociological Review* 41:262-280.

Johnson, Terence J. 1972. *Professions and Power*. London: Macmillan.

Kaufman, Martin. 1971. *Homeopathy in America: The Rise and Fall of a Medical Heresy*. Baltimore: Johns Hopkins Press.

Kendall, Patricia L. 1965. *The Relationship Between Medical Educators and Medical Practitioners.* Evanston, IL: Association of American Medical Colleges.

Kett, Joseph F. 1968. *The Formation of the American Medical Profession.* New Haven: Yale University Press.

Kronus, Carol L. 1976. "The Evolution of Occupational Power: An Historical study of Task Boundaries between Physicians and Pharmacists." *Sociology of Work and Occupations* 3(1): 3-37.

Larkin, Gerald. 1983. *Occupational Monopoly and Modern Medicine.* London: Tavistock.

Lauderdale, Pat. 1976. "Deviance and Moral Boundaries." *American Sociological Review* 41:660-76.

Law, Sylvia A. 1974. *Blue Cross - What Went Wrong?* New Haven, CT: Yale University Press.

Leis, Gordon L. 1971. "The Professionalization of Chiropractic." Ph.D. dissertation, Department of Sociology, State University of New York at Buffalo, Buffalo, NY.

Lin, Phylis Lan. 1972. "The Chiropractor, Chiropractic, and Process: A Study of the Sociology of an Occupation." Ph.D. dissertation, Department of Sociology, University of Missouri, Columbia, MO.

Litman, Theodor J. and Leonard S. Robins, eds. 1984. *Health Politics and Policy.* New York: John Wiley.

Lowes, Peter D. 1966. *The Genesis of International Narcotics Control.* Geneve: Librairie Droz.

Marmor, Theodore R. 1982. "Canada's Path, America's Choices: Lessons from the Canadian Experience with National Health Insurance." Pp. 77-96 in *Compulsory Health Insurance: The Continuing American Debate,* edited by R.L. Numbers. Westport, CT: Greenwood Press.

May, Jude Thomas, Mary L. Durham and Peter Kong-Ming New. 1980. "Professional Control and Innovation: The Neighborhood Health Center Experience." Pp. 105-136 in *Research in the Sociology of Health Care,* vol. 1, edited by J.A. Roth. Greenwich, CT: JAI Press.

Mayer, Milton. 1949. "The Rise and Fall of Dr. Fishbein." *Harpers* 199(5):76-85.

Merton, Robert K. 1949. *Social Theory and Social Structure.* Glencoe, IL: Free Press.

McKinlay, John B. and Sonja J. McKinlay. 1977. "The Questionable Contribution of Medical Measures to the Decline of Mortality in the United States in the Twentieth Century." *Milbank Memorial Fund Quarterly/Health and Society* 55(3):405-428.

Miller, A. 1977. "The Changing Structure of the Medical Profession in Urban and Suburban Settings." *Social Science and Medicine* 11(4):233-

243.

Moore, J. Stuart. 1993. *Chiropractic in America: The History of a Medical Alternative*. Baltimore: Johns Hopkin University Press.

Northwestern College of Chiropractic. 1989. *Northwestern College of Chiropractic 1989-90 General Catalog*. Bloomington, MN: Northwestern College of Chiropractic.

Plamandon, Ronald. 1993. "Summary of 1992 ACA Statistical Survey." *ACA Journal of Chiropractic* 30(2):36-42.

Quinney, Richard. 1977. *Class, State and Crime: On the Theory and Practice of Criminal Justice*. New York: David McKay.

Reed, Louis S. 1932. *The Healing Cults*, publication no. 16 of the Committee on the Costs of Medical Care. Chicago: University of Chicago Press.

Relman, Arnold. 1980. "The New Medical-Industrial Complex." *The New England Journal of Medicine* 303:963-970.

Renzetti, Claire M. and Daniel J. Curran. 1989. *Women, Men and Society*. Boston: Allyn and Bacon.

Ruzek, Sheryl Burt. 1980. "Medical Response to Women's Health Activities: Conflict Accomodation, and Cooptation." Pp. 335-354 in *Research in the Sociology of Health Care*, vol. 1, edited by J. Roth. Greenwich, CT: JAI Press.

Savo, Cynthia. 1983. "Self-Care and Empowerment." *Social Policy* 14(1):9-22.

Schwartz, Howard D. and Ian Siederman. 1987. "Lay Initiatives in the Consumption of Health Care." Pp. 221-235 in *Dominant Issues in Medical Sociology*, 2d ed., edited by H. S. Schwartz. New York: Random House.

Shryock, Richard Harrison. 1967. *Medical Licensing in America 1650-1965*. Baltimore: The Johns Hopkins Press.

------. [1936] 1974. *The Development of Modern Medicine: An Interpretation of the Social and Scientific Factors Involved*. Madison, WI: University of Wisconsin Press.

Smith, Harvey L. 1955. "Two Lines of Authority Are One Too Many." *Modern Hospital* 84:59-64.

Stanford Research Institute. 1960. *Chiropractic in California*. Los Angeles: Haynes Foundation.

Starr, Paul. 1982. *The Social Transformation of American Medicine*. New York: Basic Books.

Turner, Chittenden. 1931. *The Rise of Chiropractic*. Los Angeles: Powell Publishing Co.

U.S. Department of Health, Education and Welfare. 1978. "Utilization of

Selected Medical Practitioners: United States 1974." *Advance Data: Vital and Health Statistics of the National Center for Health Statistics* No. 24(March 24):1-3.

------. 1966. "Chiropractor." *National Center for Health Statistics*, Series 10, 28(May):37.

Vogl, A.J. 1974. "It's Time to Take Chiropractors Seriously." *Medical Economics* 51(Dec. 9):76-85.

Vold, George B. 1958. *Theoretical Criminology*. New York: Oxford University Press.

Von Kuster, Jr., Thomas. 1980. *Chiropractic Health Care*, vol. I. Washington, D.C.: Foundation for the Advancement of Chiropractic Tenets and Science.

Wardwell, Walter I. 1992. *Chiropractic: History and Evolution of a New Profession*. St. Louis, MO: Mosby-Yearbook, Inc.

------. 1982. "Chiropractors: Challengers of Medical Domination." Pp.207-250 in *Research in the Sociology of Health Care*, vol. 2, edited by J.A. Roth. Greenwich, CT: JAI Press.

------. 1963. "Limited, Marginal, and Quasi-Practitioners." Pp. 213-239 in *Handbook of Medical Sociology*, edited by H. Freeman, S. Levine, and L. Reeder. Englewood Cliffs, NJ: Prentice-Hall.

------. 1951. "Social Strain and Social Adjustment in the Marginal Role of the Chiropractor." Ph.D. dissertation, Department of Social Relations, Harvard University, Cambridge, MA.

Weber, Max. [1904]1949. *The Methodology of the Social Sciences*. translated and edited by Edward A. Shills and Henry A. Finch. NY: Free Press.

Weiant, C.W. and S. Goldschmidt. 1966. *What Medicine Really Thinks about Chiropractic: A Study in Conflict*. Des Moines, IA: American Chiropractic Association.

Wertz, Richard W. and Dorothy C. Wertz. 1977. *Lying In: A History of Childbirth in America*. NY: Macmillan.

Withorn, Ann. 1986. "Helping Ourselves." Pp. 416-424 in *The Sociology of Health and Illness*, 2d ed., edited by P. Conrad and R. Kern. New York: St. Martin's Press.

Wolinsky, Fredric D. and William D. Marder. 1985. *The Organization of Medcial Practice and the Practice of Medicine*. Ann Arbor, MI: Health Administration Press.

Index